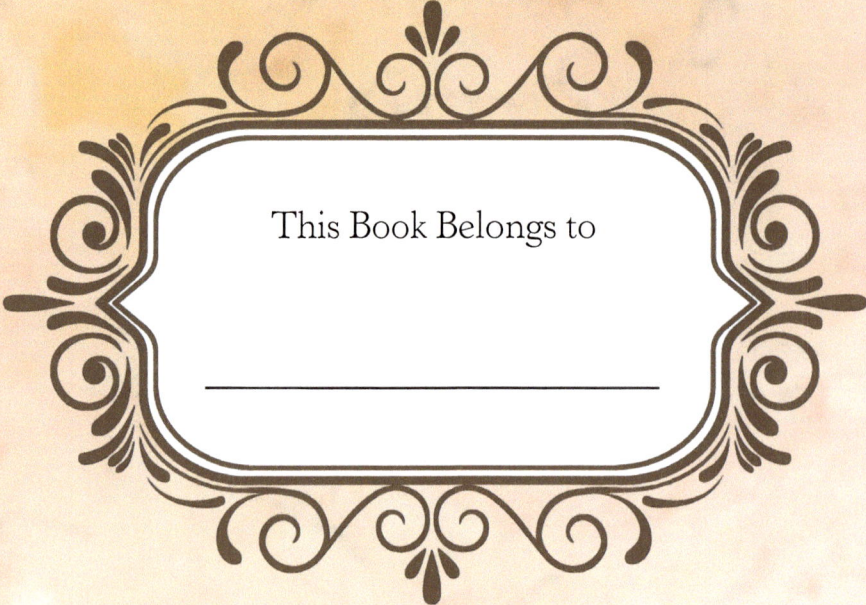

This Book Belongs to

_____

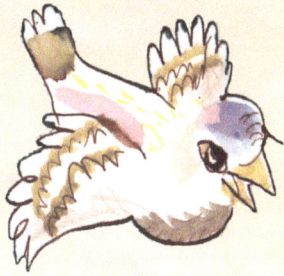

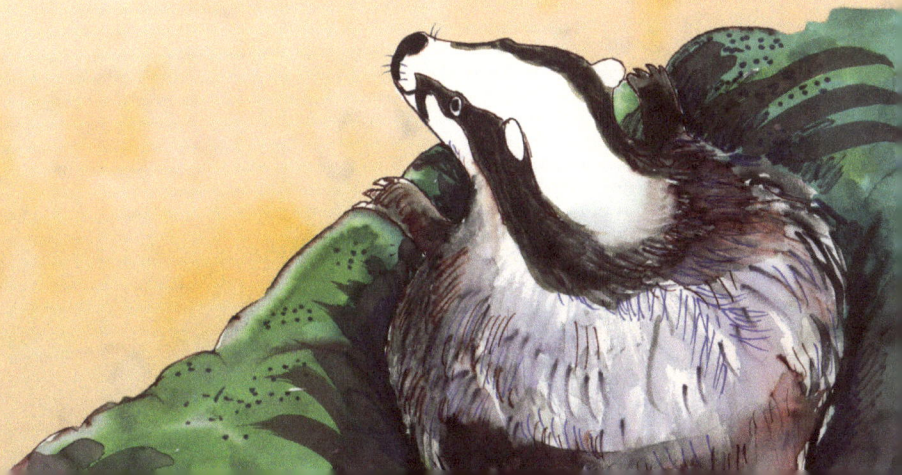

Martina and the Ogre

Author - Frank Kinslow

Illustrator - Mirek Raboch

Book Design - Angel Navarro

Book Editor - Barbara Vesey

Production Editor - Martina Kinslow

Library of Congress Control Number: 2014914408

LucidSea

ISBN 978-0-9844264-3-0

Martina
and the
Ogre

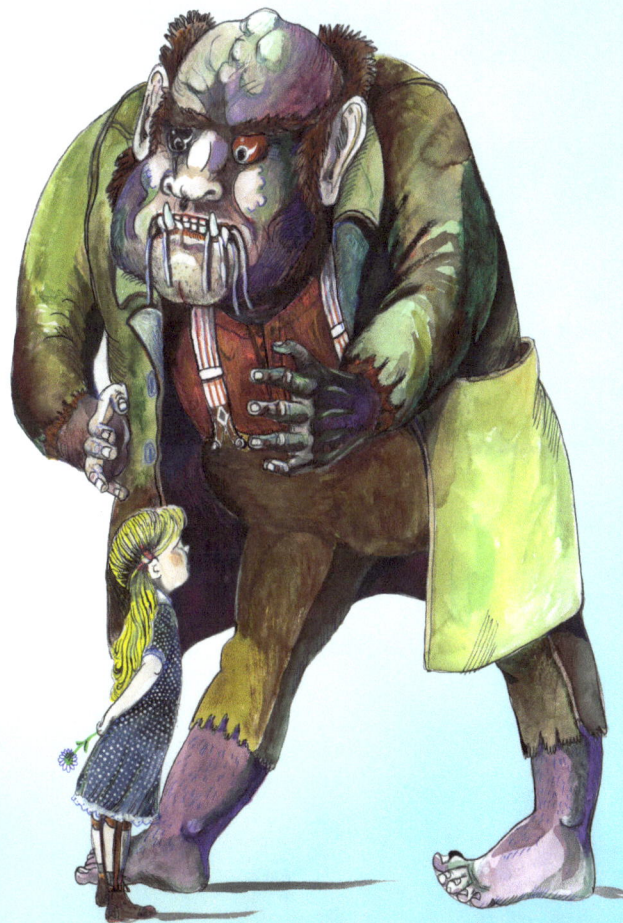

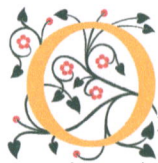

Once upon a time there was a little village nestled just on the other side of a hill from a beautiful blue lake. There was a long, long wooden bridge that went from one side of the lake all the way over to the other side. It was so far that no one could see the other end of the long, long bridge.

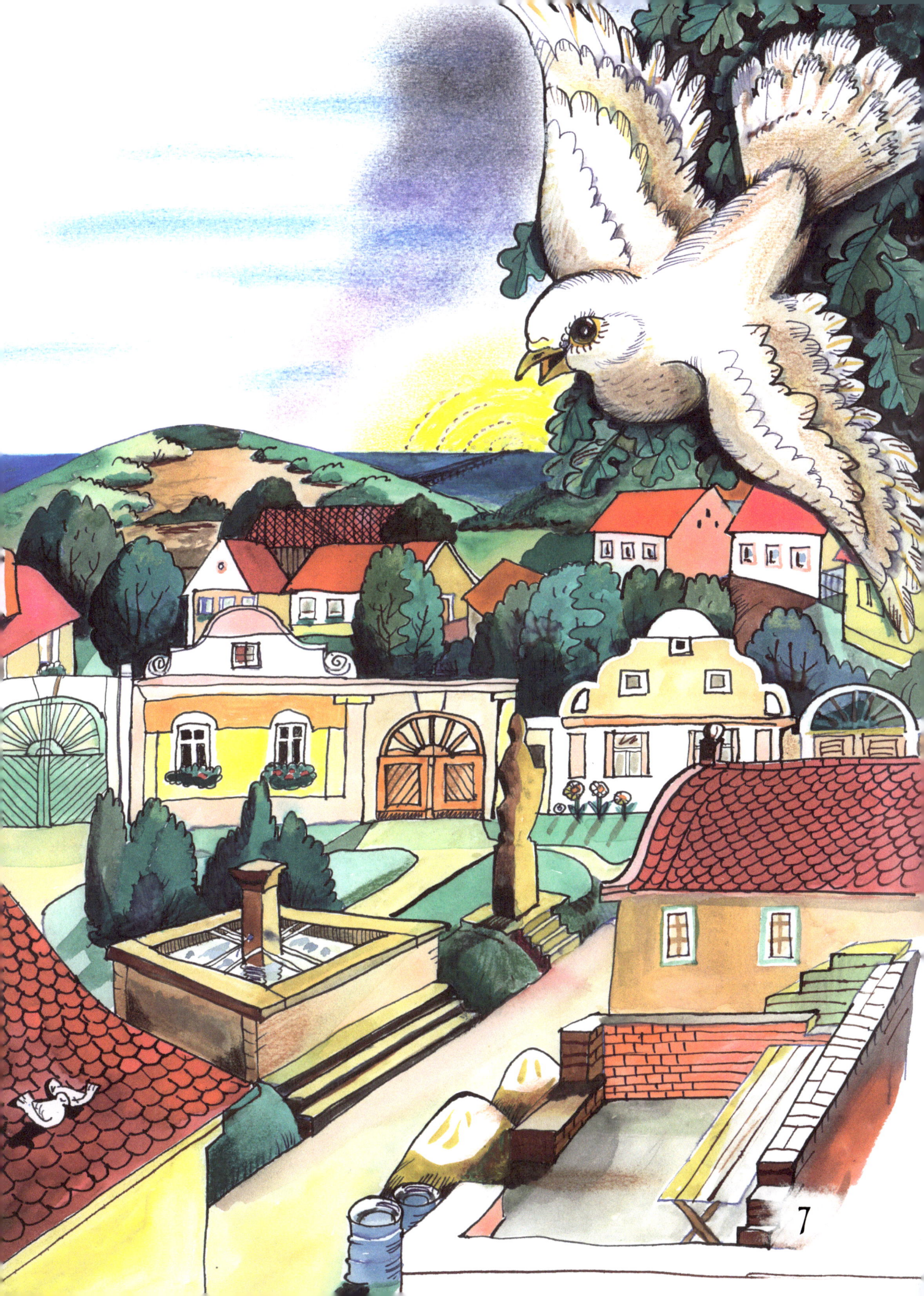

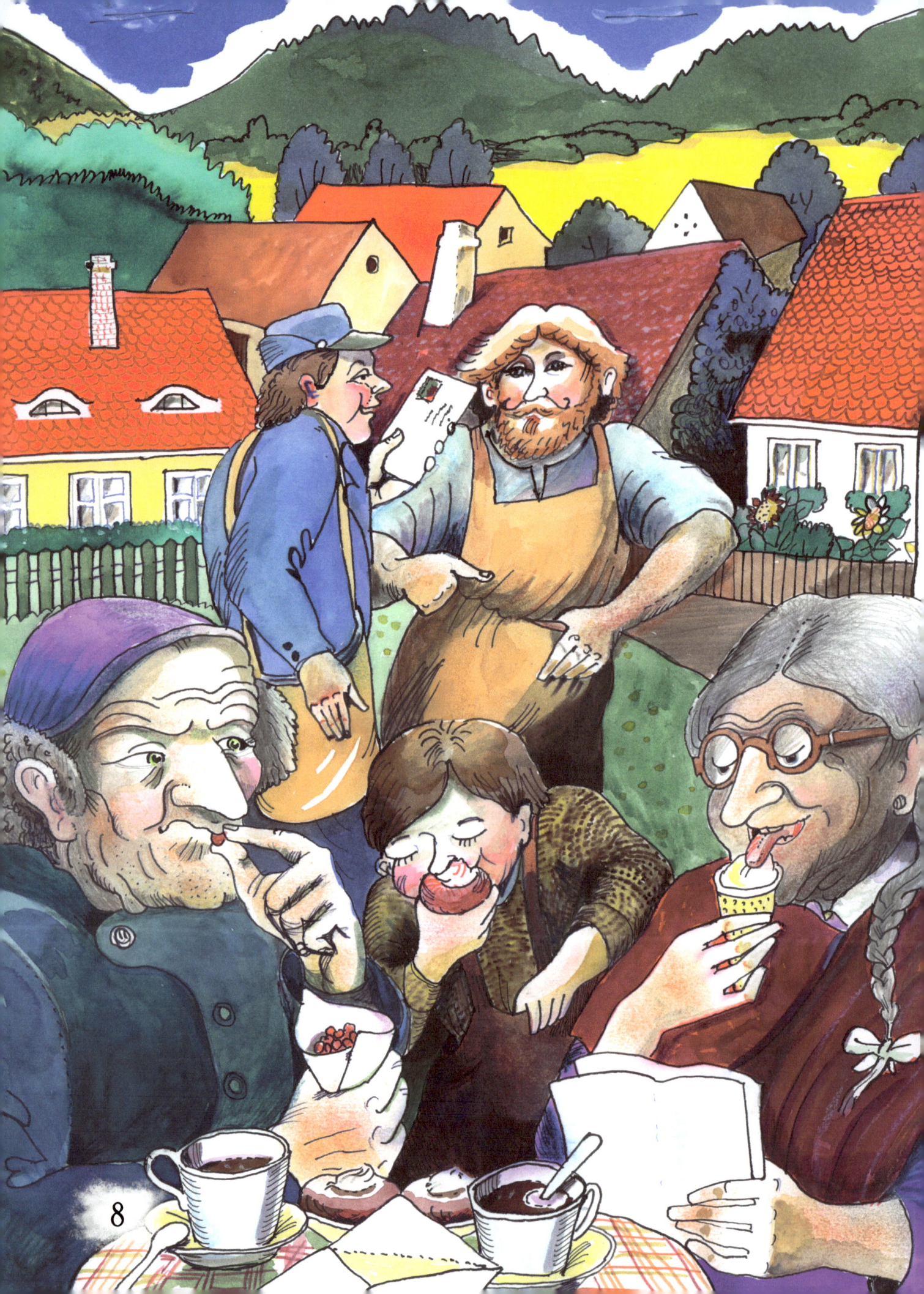

The people of the village were always very busy.

— "What did they do?"

Why, all sorts of important things—like delivering mail and building houses and writing down lots and lots of numbers to keep track of everything. They also ate lots of tasty foods, including doughnuts, cupcakes, and ice cream. They especially loved ice cream—I think rum raisin was their favorite.

Every Sunday the people of the busy little village would meet in the town square under the wide oak tree and talk about the beautiful blue lake just over the hill from the town.

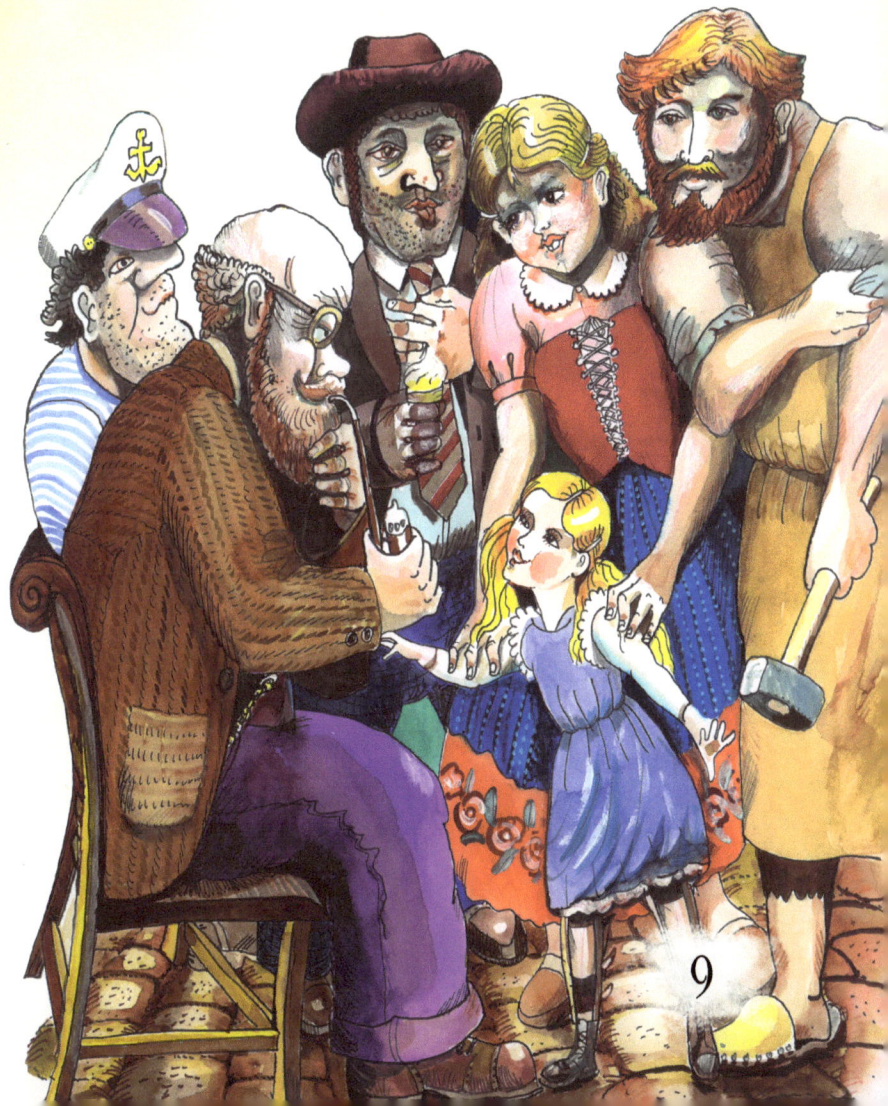

9

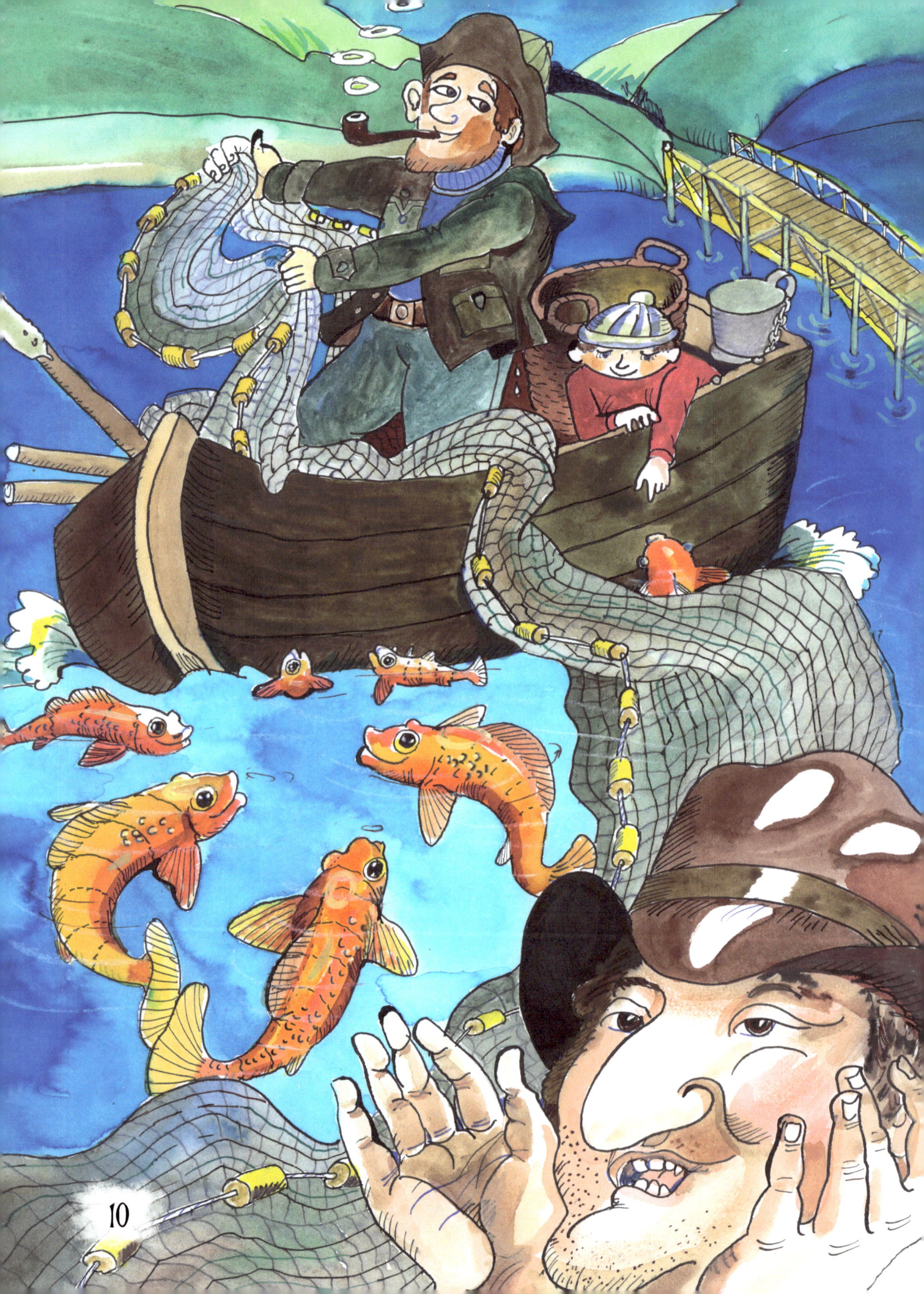

Some would tell stories about men who had visited the lake many years before and had described how beautiful it really was.

They said how clear and deep the lake was, and that laughing rainbow-colored catfish would swim right up to their boat, roll over, and ask them to pet their soft little bellies.

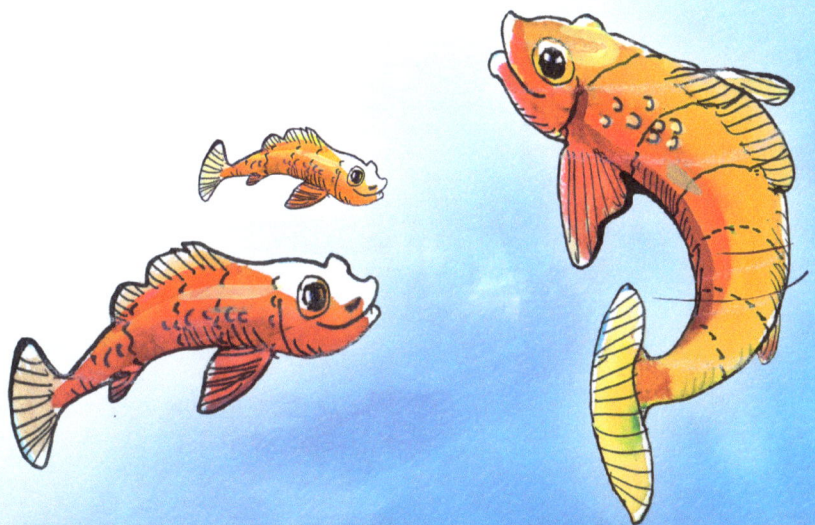

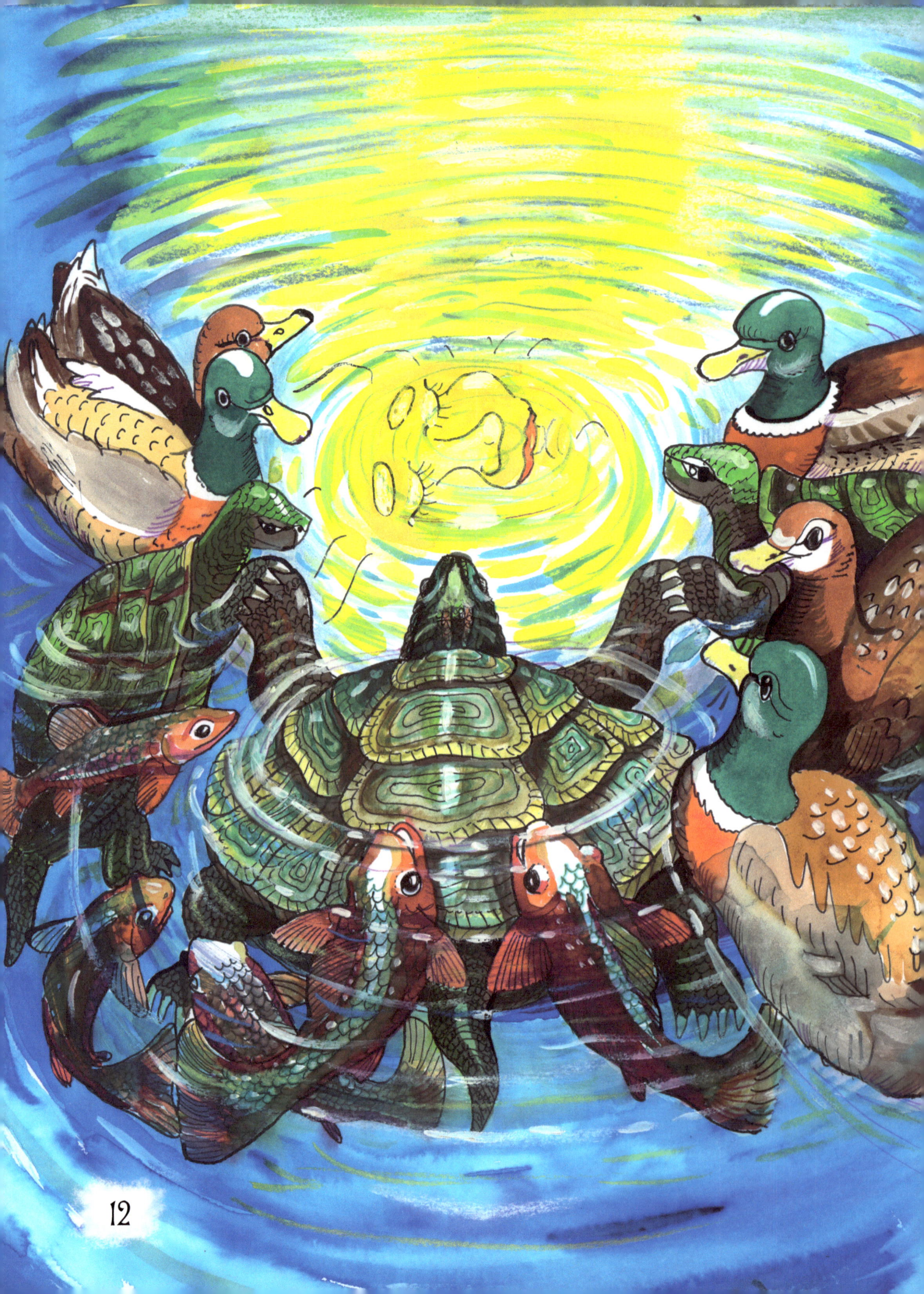

They told tales of how the ducks and turtles would sing a song to the sun while dogfish barked and wagged their tales in time to the music.

The people of the busy little village were happy on Sundays when they talked about the lake. But the very next day, and all through the week, they forgot all about it and went back to the worries of being busy.

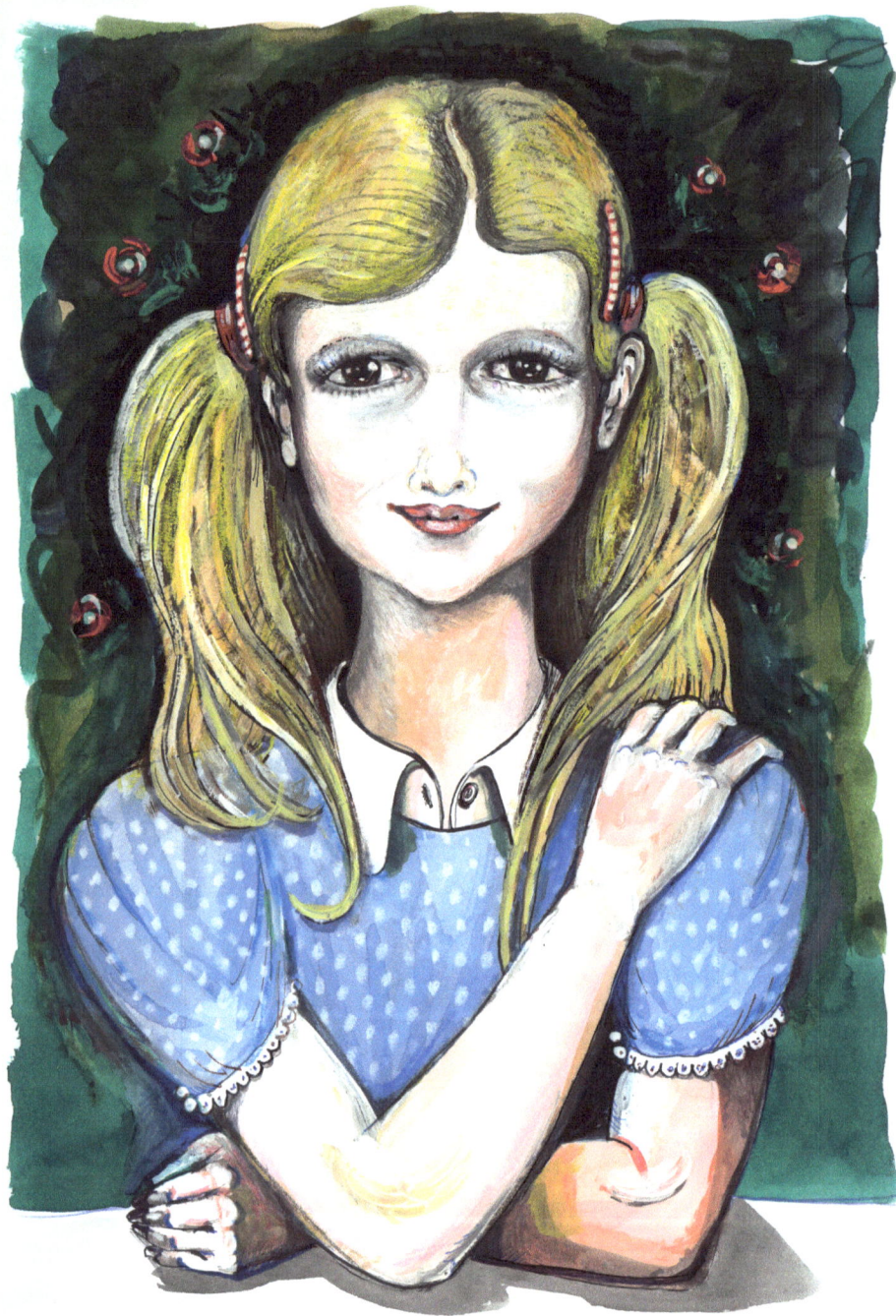

In the busy little village, there lived a quietly happy girl named Sweet Little Martina. She had lovely blonde hair that flowed and swung around her shoulders whenever she turned her head. Her deep brown eyes glistened like water in sunshine whenever they were open, and probably did so when they were closed as well.

Sweet Little Martina had tiny wooden braces to help her walk because her legs were very, very weak. But she didn't seem to notice much, for she would play with the other children of the busy little village from sun-up to sundown. She never complained or said it was unfair that she couldn't run or jump like the other children.

Sweet Little Martina always greeted everybody with a big smile and happiness in her voice.

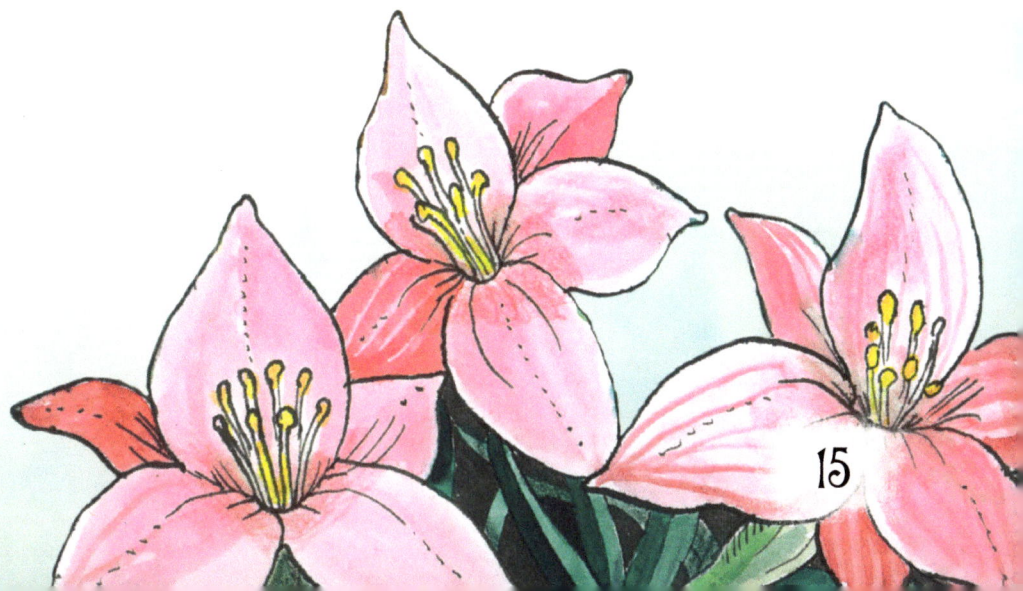

One reason why Sweet Little Martina was so happy was because her mother and father had taught her how to go to her secret happy place. It was a special place that all children have inside them. It is always there on sunny days but you have to look for it on cloudy days.

Once she learned to go to her happy place she was rarely ever afraid. And if she ever became fearful of a really, really bad storm with scary flashes of lightning and loud thunder, or if she thought that a monster was hiding under her bed, she would recall what her parents had taught her. Martina would just let her thoughts go to that happy place inside her and the scary parts would all go away. It even made the hurt in her legs vanish.

And if she fell and scraped her hands and knees —as she would sometimes do when playing with the other children—she'd simply do what her father and mother had taught her and the pain would stop.

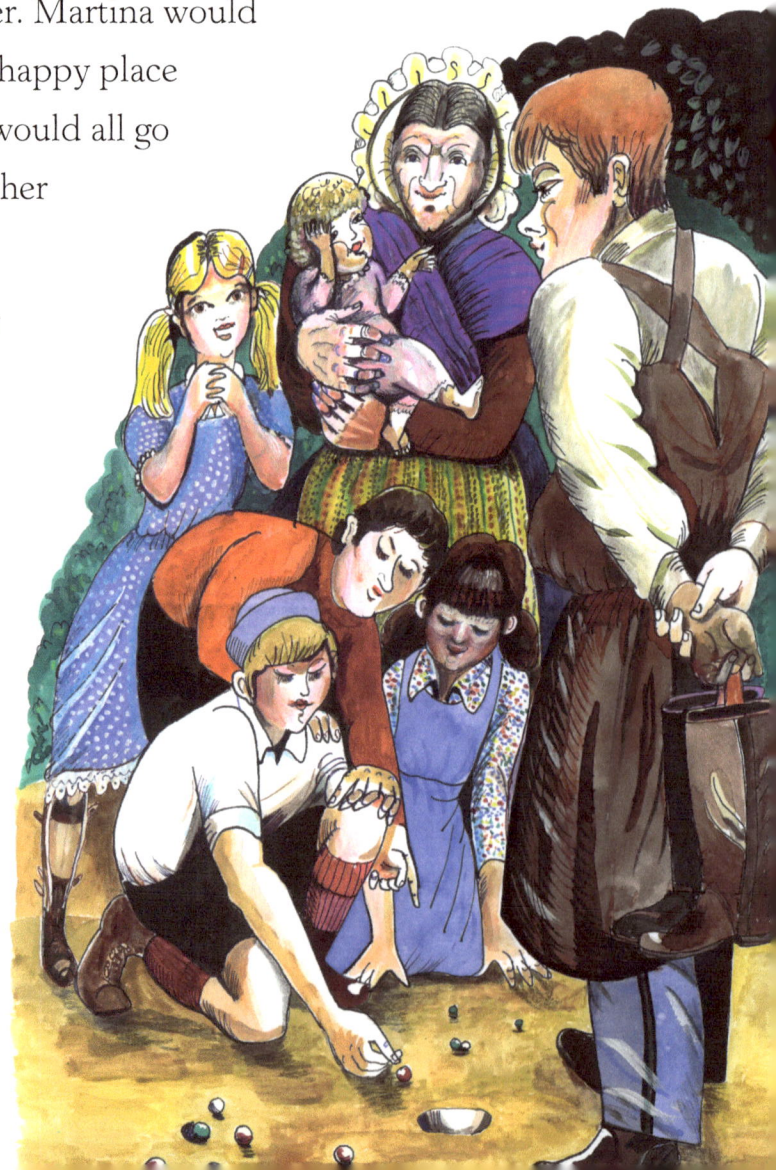

She loved her happy place and would even go there when her legs weren't hurting or when she wasn't afraid. Her happy place was the reason why people said she had sunrise eyes.

Every morning Sweet Little Martina would sit in front of her mirror and brush her hair. While she brushed her hair she sang this hair-brushing song:

— "Diddly-doo Diddly-dee,
won't you please look at me?"

— "I'm a big girl, as you can see. I brush my hair down to my knee."

— "Diddly-doo Diddly-dee,
Diddly, diddly, diddly-dee."

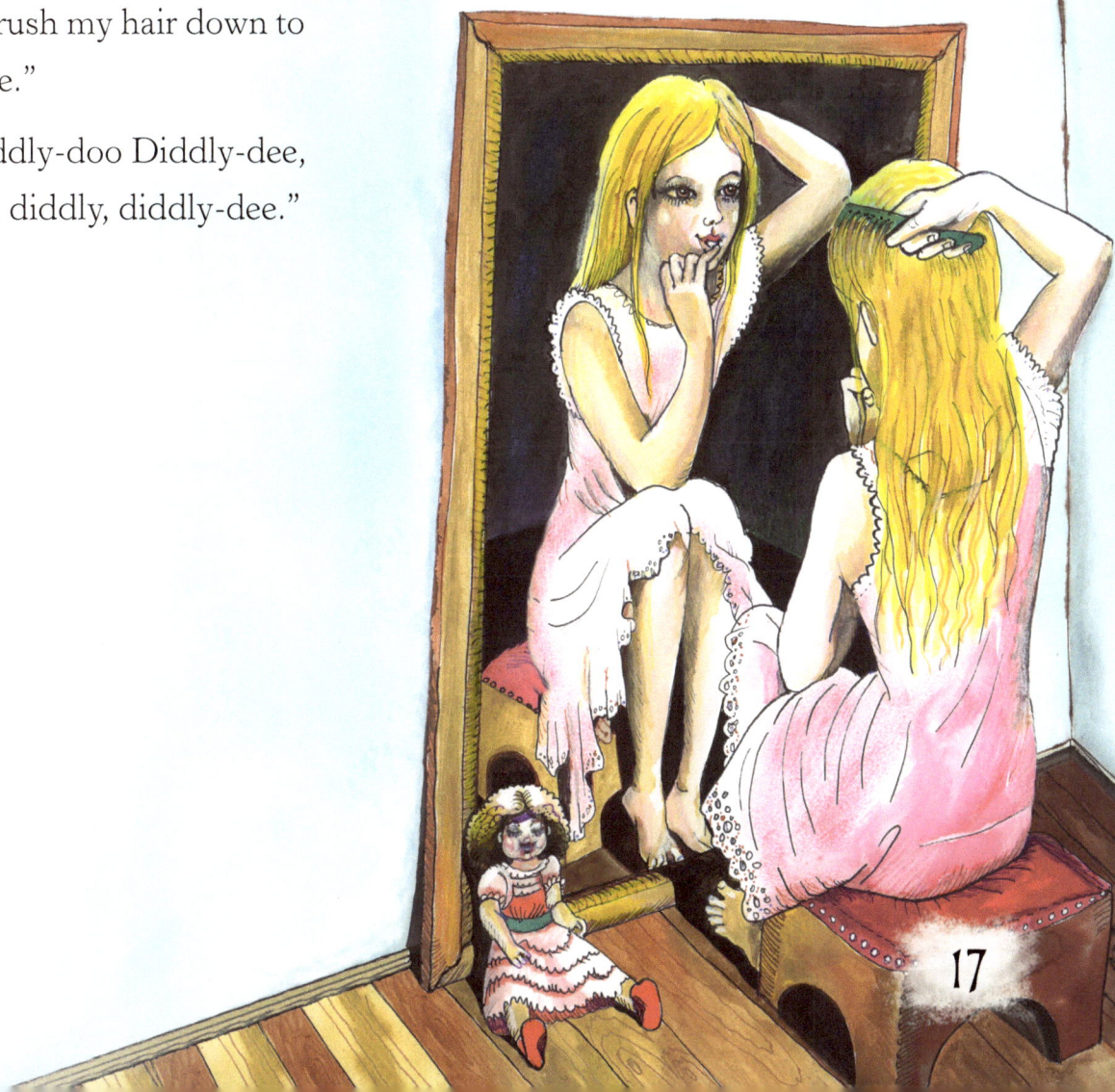

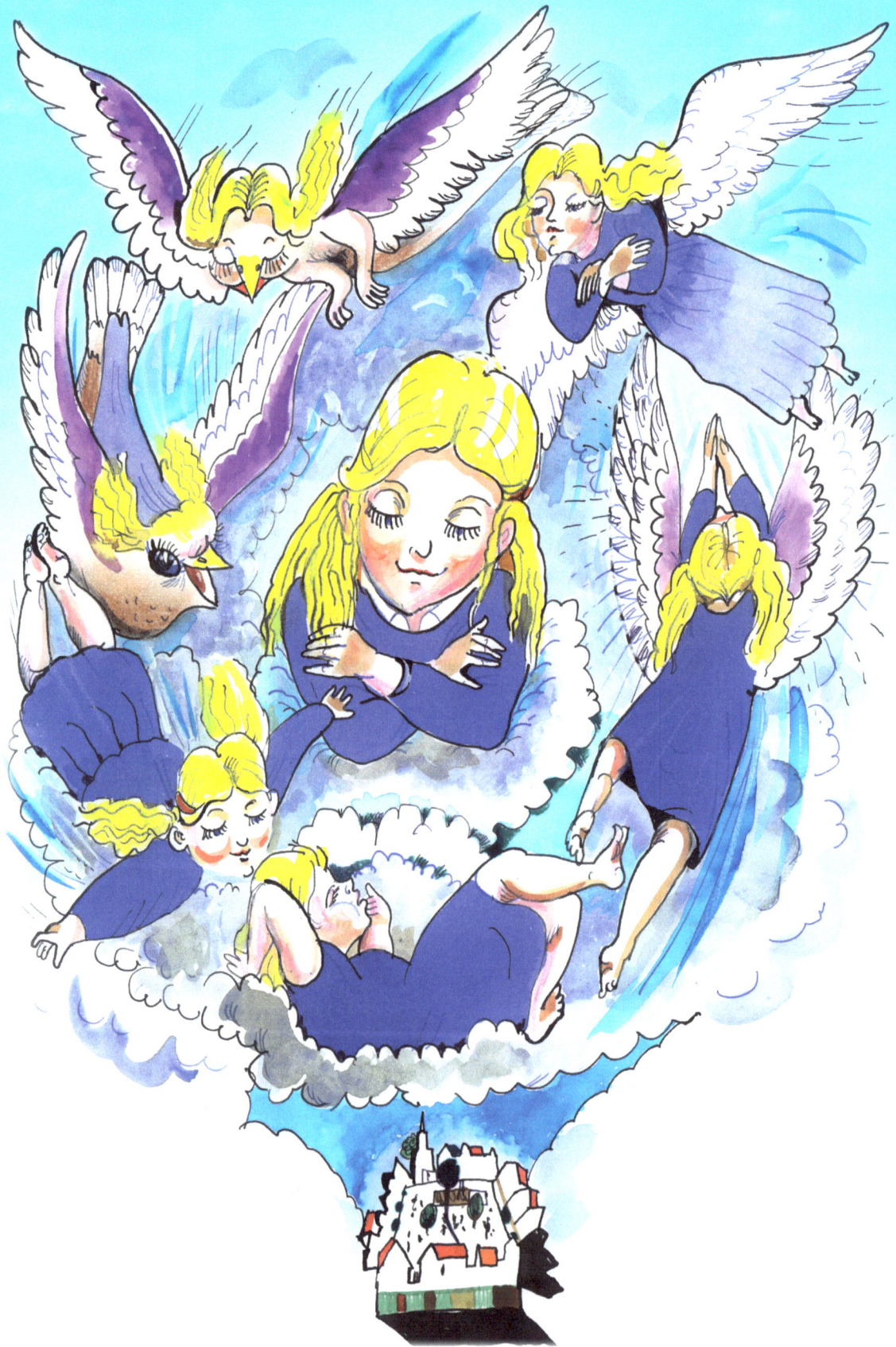

Sweet Little Martina was very polite and very, very inquisitive. She loved to ask questions. Sometimes she would ask,

— "Where do clouds come from?" or

— "What is at the end of all the numbers?" or

— "Why can't I fly like the birds do?"

If she could, she would fly high up in the sky with her arms stretched way out; and when she got tired, she would lie down on a fluffy white cloud and watch all the people of the busy little village as they scampered around like wee little ants on a sugar cube.

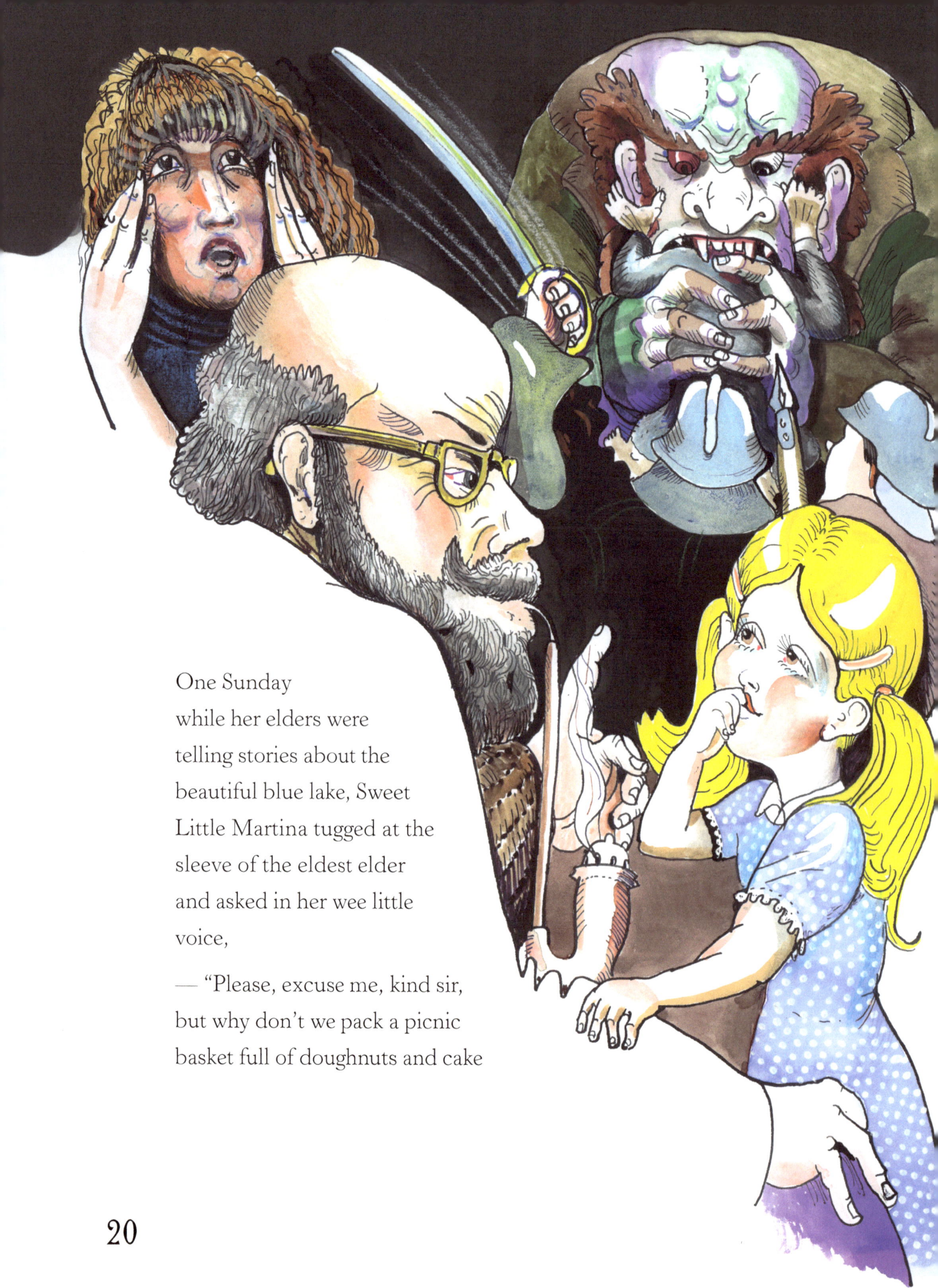

One Sunday
while her elders were
telling stories about the
beautiful blue lake, Sweet
Little Martina tugged at the
sleeve of the eldest elder
and asked in her wee little
voice,

— "Please, excuse me, kind sir,
but why don't we pack a picnic
basket full of doughnuts and cake

and bottles of cherry root beer (which tickles your nose when you drink it) and have a picnic by the side of the beautiful blue lake?"

A hush fell over the townspeople, and they looked very serious indeed. The eldest elder finally spoke, saying,

— "We can never go to the beautiful blue lake, for under the long, long bridge lives an evil ogre."

He told Sweet Little Martina that they never spoke about the ogre because they didn't want to scare the little children, but he was twice as tall as a man and as big around as the big oak tree in the village square that they were sitting under that very moment.

His skin was purple with green spots, and it was slimy and smelly and bumpy. He had jagged green teeth with strings of old spaghetti hanging down because he never brushed after meals. He was a very naughty ogre. His breath smelled like tuna fish and broccoli and dirty socks all mixed together.

The ogre had one red eye and one black eye, and could see where he'd been without turning around. That's why you could never sneak up from behind to catch him. Many brave men and women had tried, and no one knows where they are now. His name was Ego the Ogre.

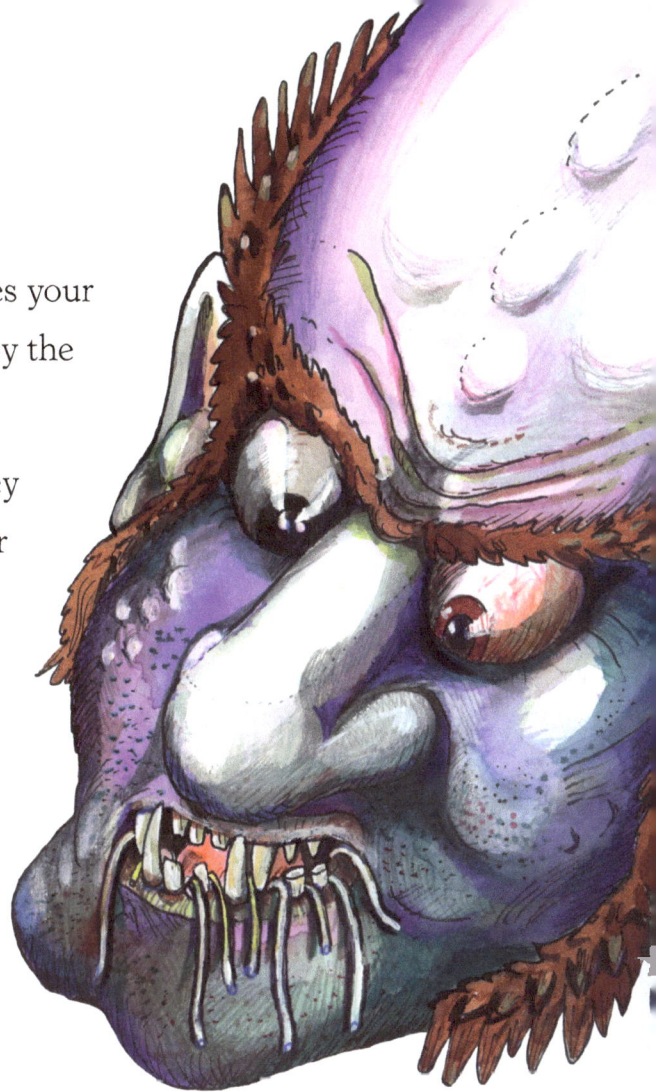

21

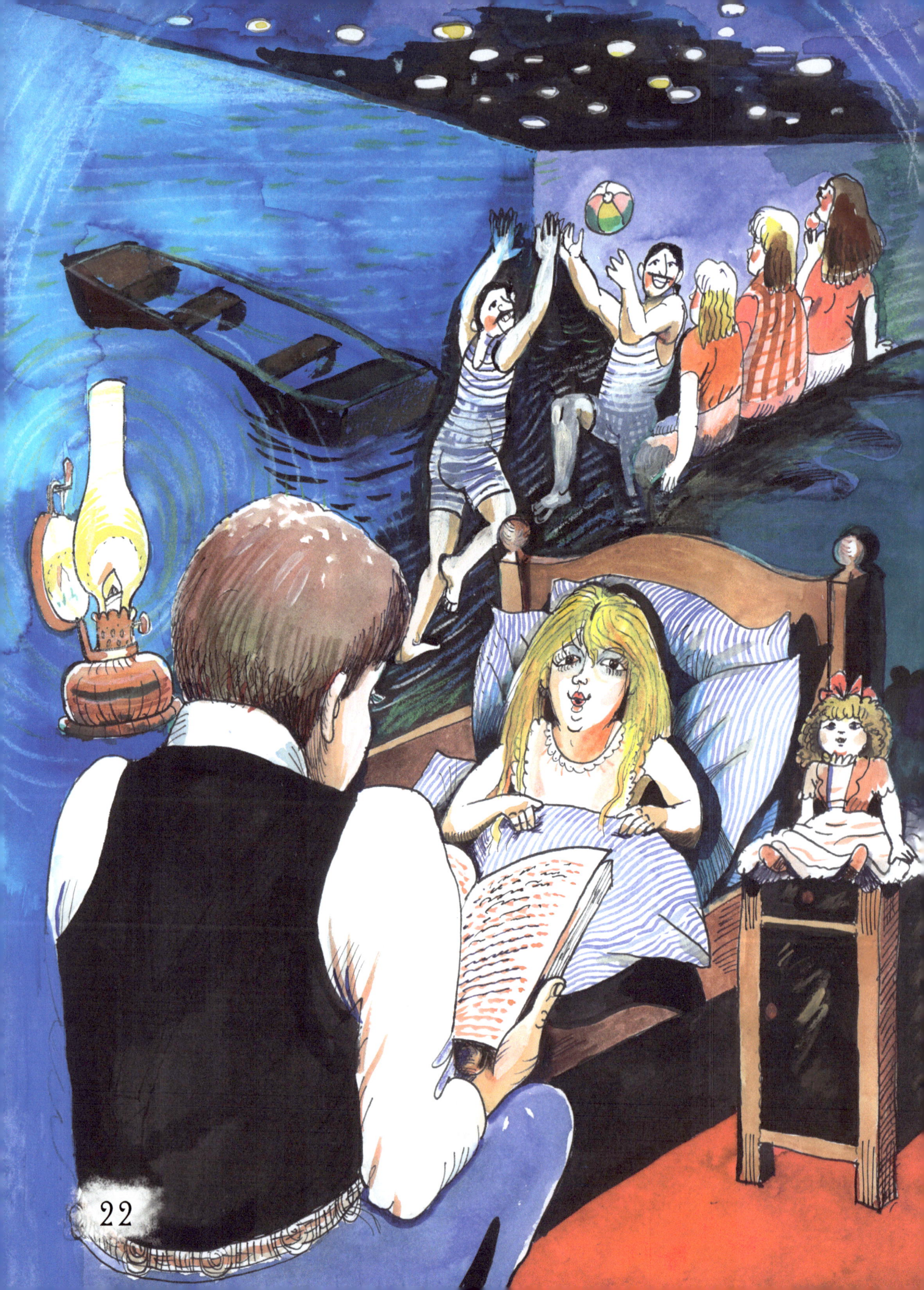

That night Sweet Little Martina listened as her father read her a bedtime story about the good old days on the beautiful blue lake before Ego the Ogre came to live under the bridge. Sweet Little Martina wanted it to be that way again so that all the people of the busy little village could go on a wonderful picnic by the side of the beautiful blue lake.

So as soon as the rooster crowed and the sun peeked its shiny, bright eye over the Long-way-away Mountains, Martina slipped out of bed, quiet as a mouse, and put on her outside clothes.

She strapped her braces to her legs and laced up her shoes, then slipped quietly outside, making sure not to slam the door.

She raised her chin, took a deep breath, and started out for the long, long bridge over the beautiful blue lake on the other side of the hill at the edge of town.

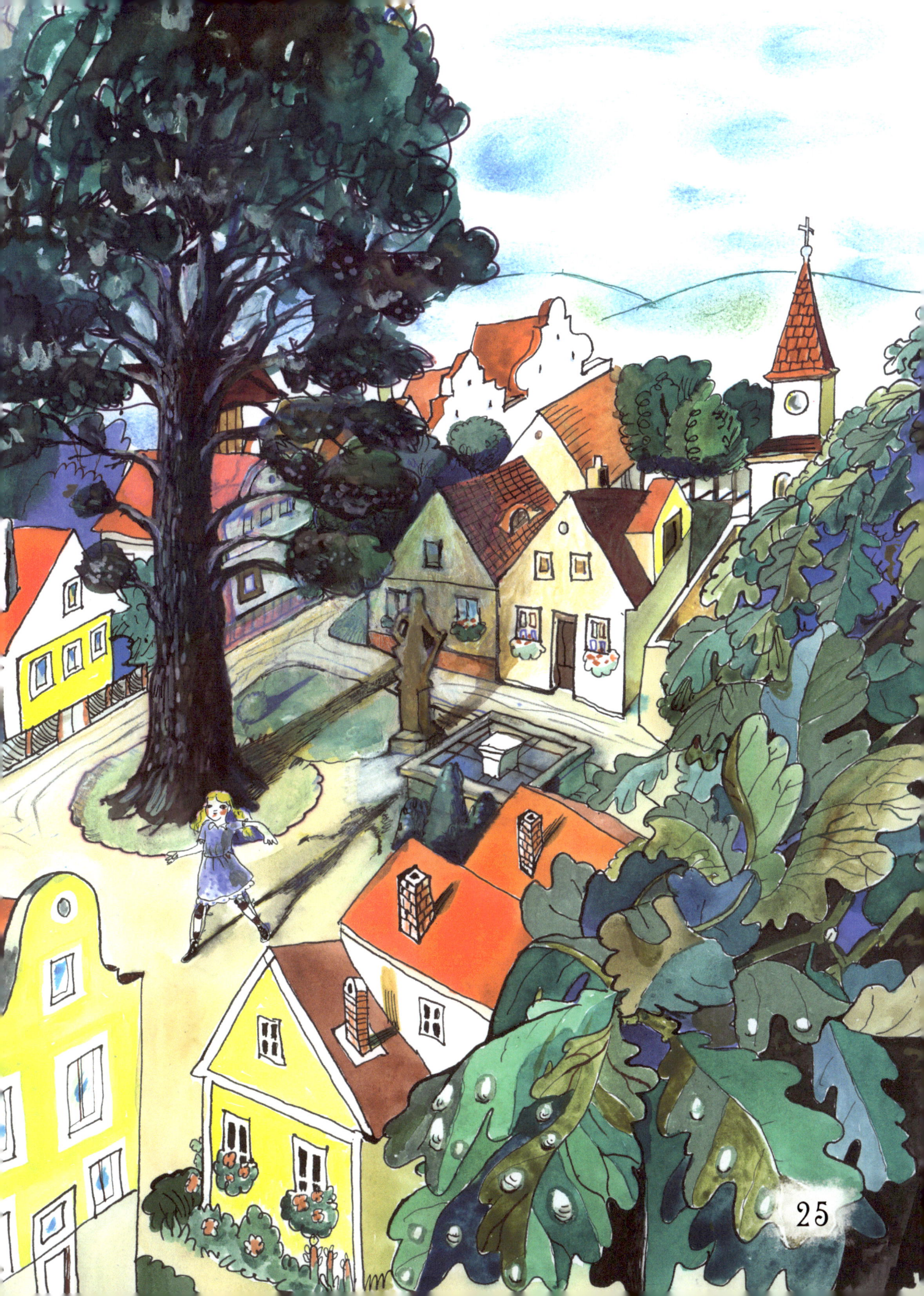

On her way, she listened to the birds singing to their babies in the nest:

— "Get up, get up, you sleepy heads."

— "Shake your little tail feathers and open your beaks."

— "It's time for your wiggly breakfast worms."

— "With marmalade and day-old leeks."

She giggled at the laughter of the leaves in the trees that were tickled by the morning breeze as it brushed against their bellies. By the side of the field where the old badger lived, she bent over and picked a single sunshine daisy, and then she skipped down the dirt road all the way to the long, long bridge.

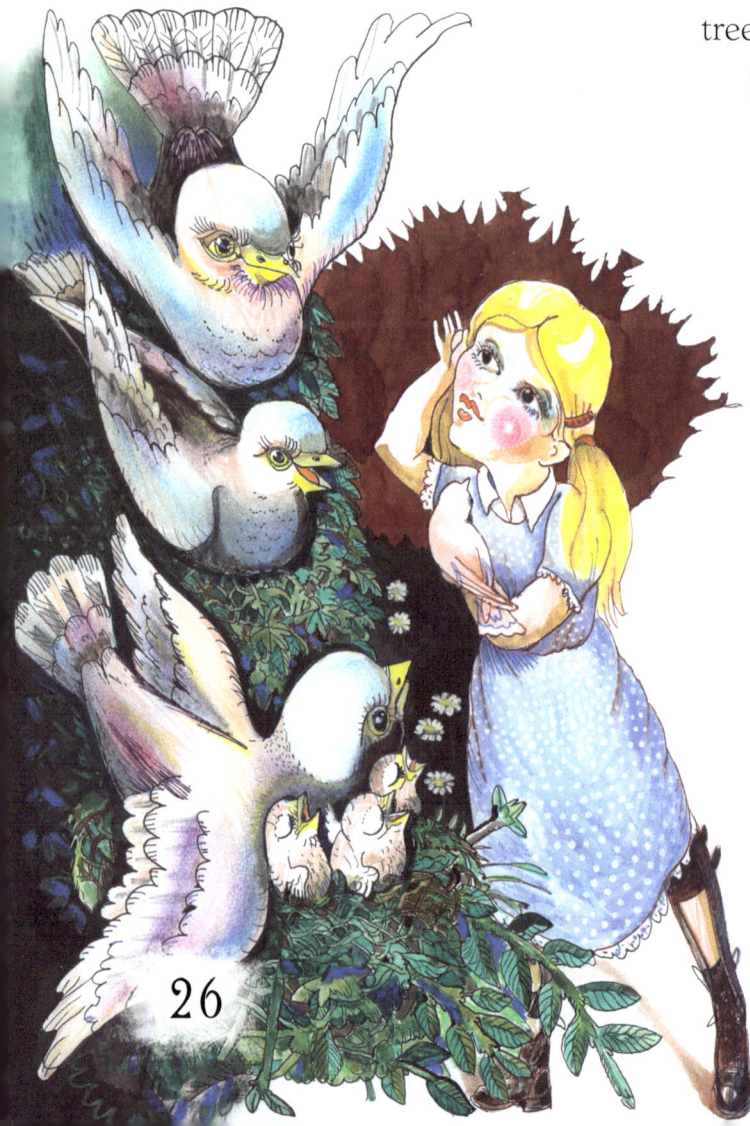

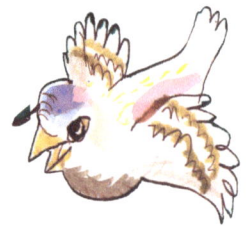

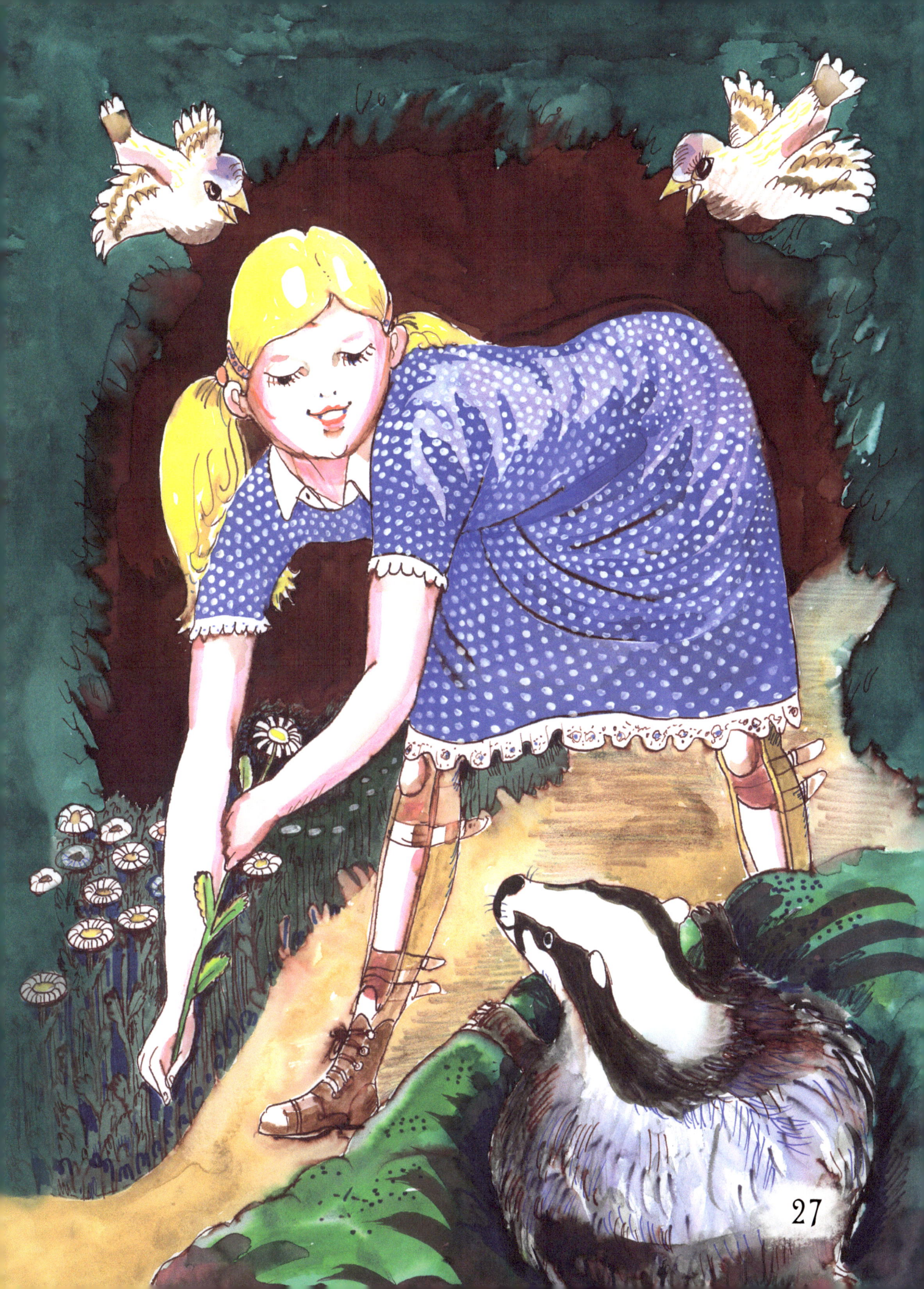

When she got to the long, long bridge, Sweet Little Martina stopped and listened and looked, just like you do before crossing a street where cars go by.

Everything was quite peaceful. She thought that maybe Ego the Ogre had met another ogre and had gotten married under the tall, tall bridge in the big, busy city beyond the Long-way-away Mountains. She thought that maybe they moved under a respectable bridge in a good neighborhood where they could raise a family of two little ogres and own a pet rumplededumpleshnick— an ogre's best friend.

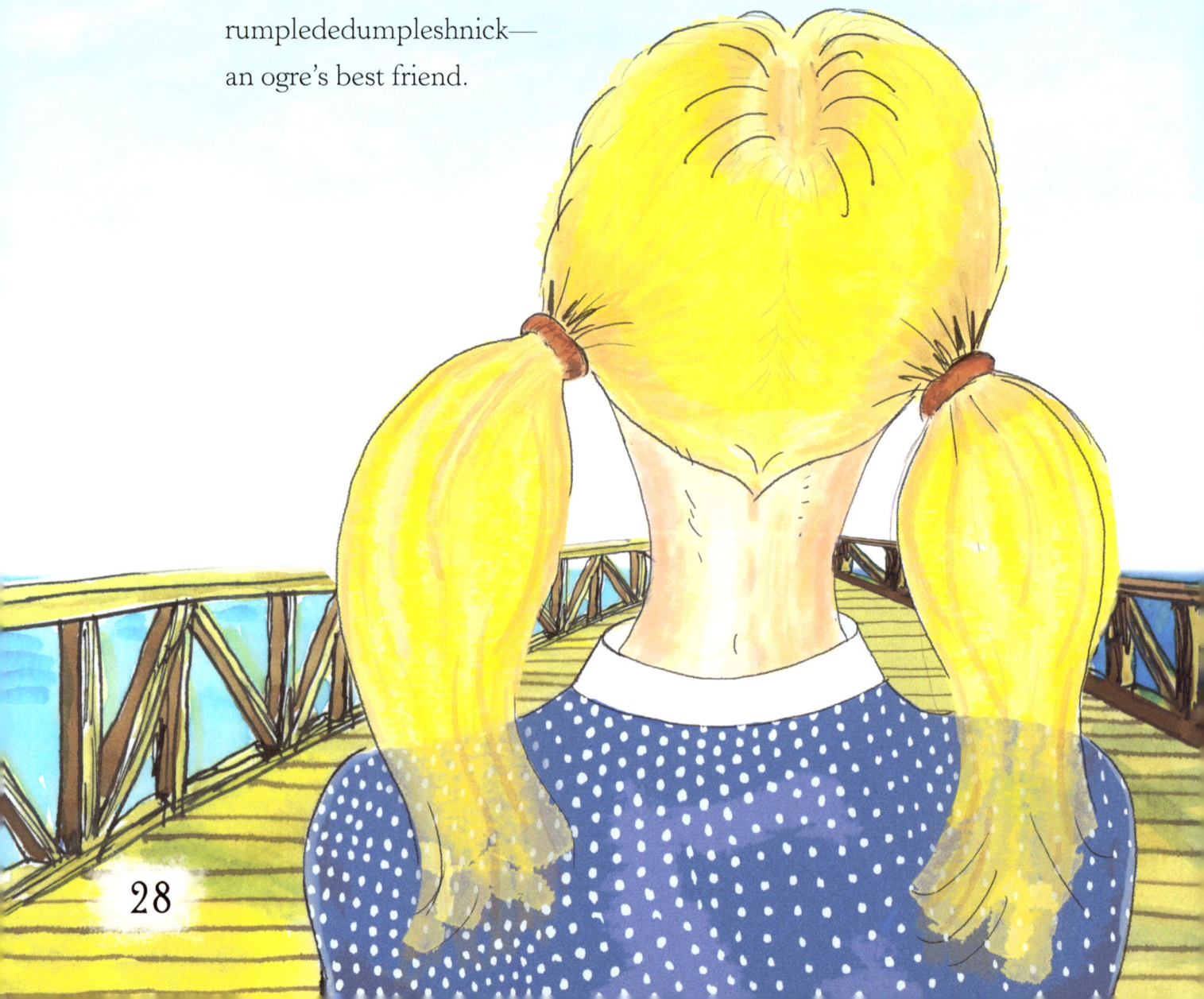

She walked slowly and quietly up to the end of the long, long bridge and waited. Nothing. Then she looked way across the long, long bridge, but couldn't see the other side, so she stepped forward.

As soon as her tiny tippy toe touched the first step on the bridge, she heard a deep, rolling grumble like thunder coming from a dark basement. The bridge shook and swayed, but the water beneath stayed calm and clear. Instead of running away, Sweet Little Martina (did I mention that she was very brave?) said in her wee little voice,

— "Who's that under the bridge?"

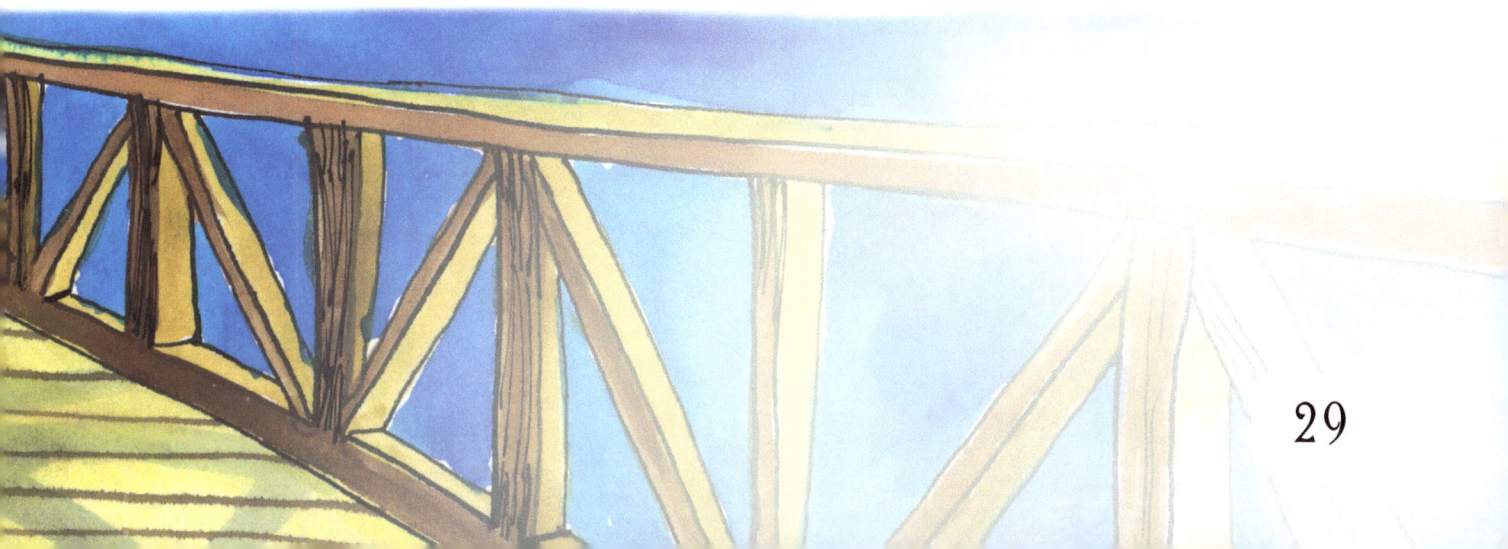

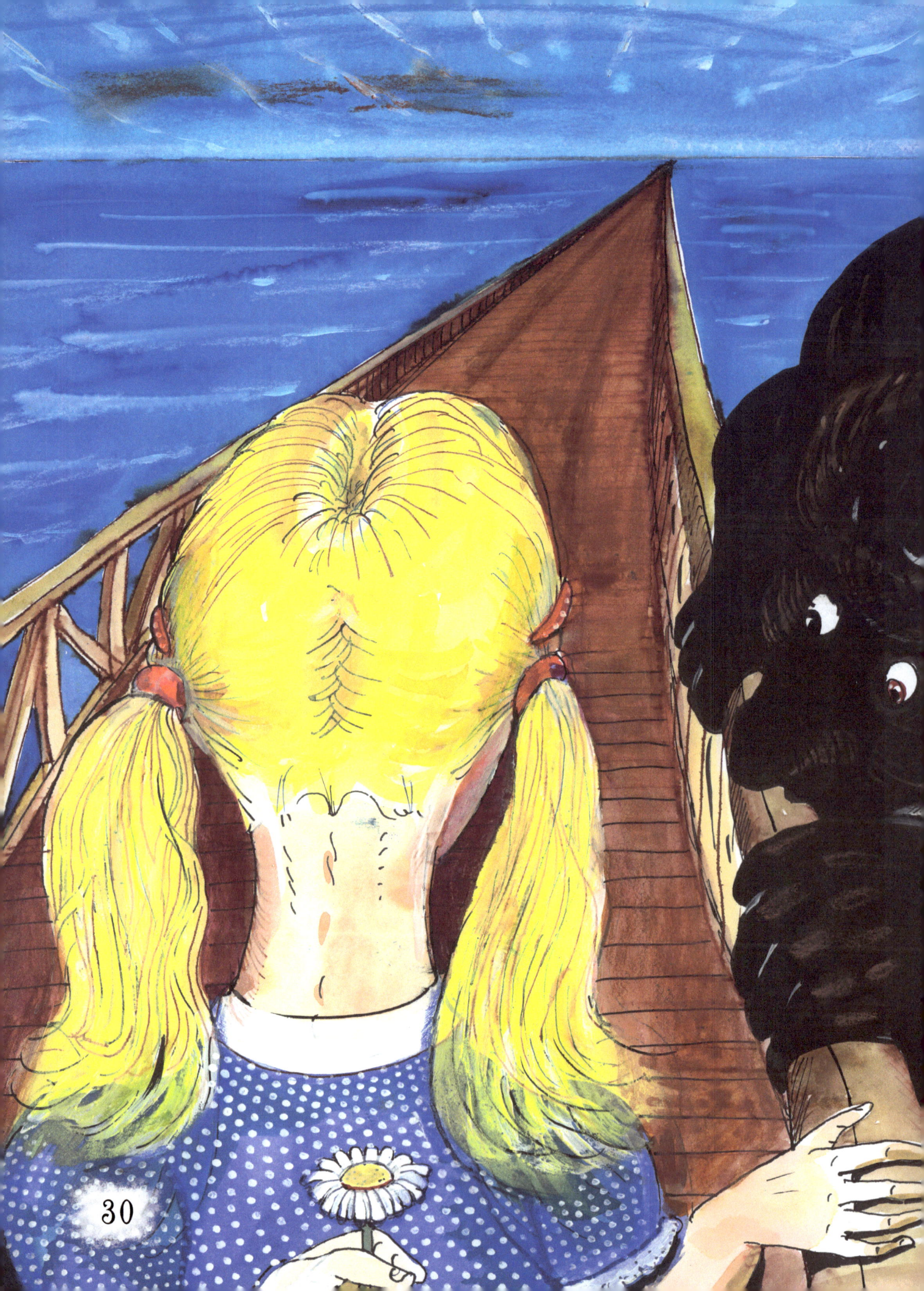

The grumble grew louder, and then she heard a grumpy voice:

— "It is I, Ego the Ogre. Do you want me to eat you up?"

— "No!" Sweet Little Martina replied with a shiver. "I only want to introduce myself and say hello."

— "Go away before I have you with my breakfast of snakes and sawdust—and, of course, my one-a-day muti-vitamin."

Sweet Little Martina was very afraid, but she remembered to go to her Happy Place, and then she wasn't afraid anymore. She stood her ground and said in a pretend angry voice,

— "I will not leave until you come out and greet me like a proper gentleman!"

The bridge shook more violently this time, and Ego the Ogre's voice boomed and bounced off the Long-way-away Mountains into the faraway lands beyond the village. All the villagers heard the noise and came out of their houses in their nightgowns with cups of coffee sloshing on the ground, except the farmer who had been up for hours milking his cows. Everyone had nervous looks on their faces and worried tones in their voices.

Then Sweet Little Martina's father and mother came running out of the house, crying,

— "Oh where, oh where can our Sweet Little Martina be? She's not in her bed, and she has had no breakfast."

Immediately the townspeople began looking all over their village for Sweet Little Martina, but she was nowhere to be found.

Then the eldest elder said,

— "I think she has gone to the long, long bridge across the beautiful blue lake over the hill that is at the edge of our village."

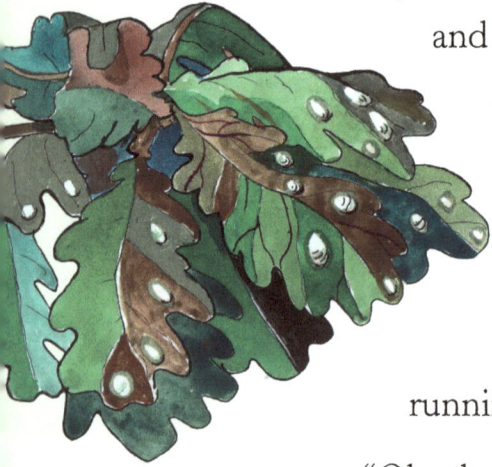

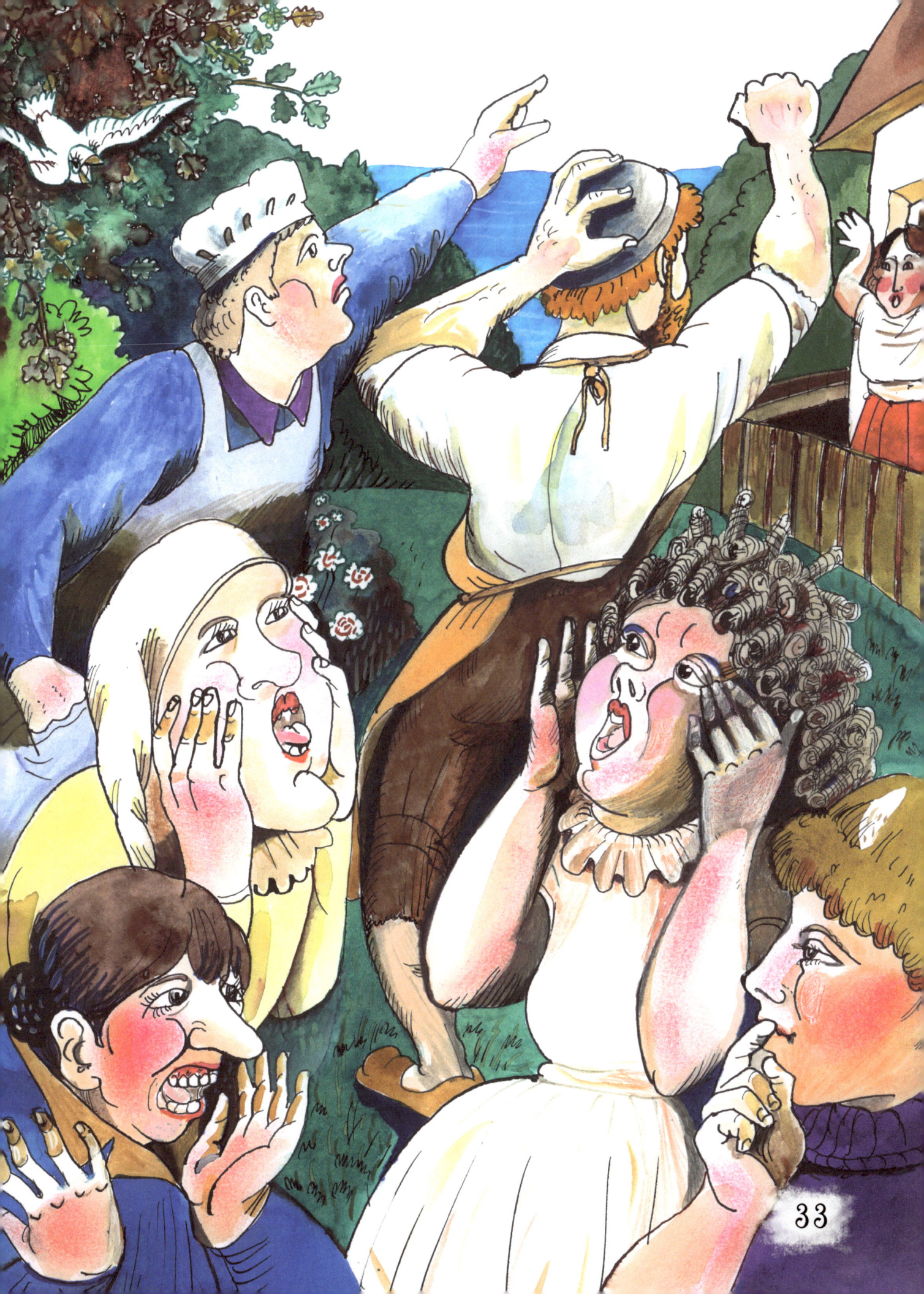

The others agreed, and they gathered every weapon they could find. They got brooms and tennis rackets and willow branches and boxing gloves. One man even took the wobbly old sword from the statue of Horace the Ogre Slayer, which stood in the town square next to the wide oak tree.

While the town's residents were arming themselves and deciding who should be in the front of the line to rescue Sweet Little Martina, she was dealing with her own problems.

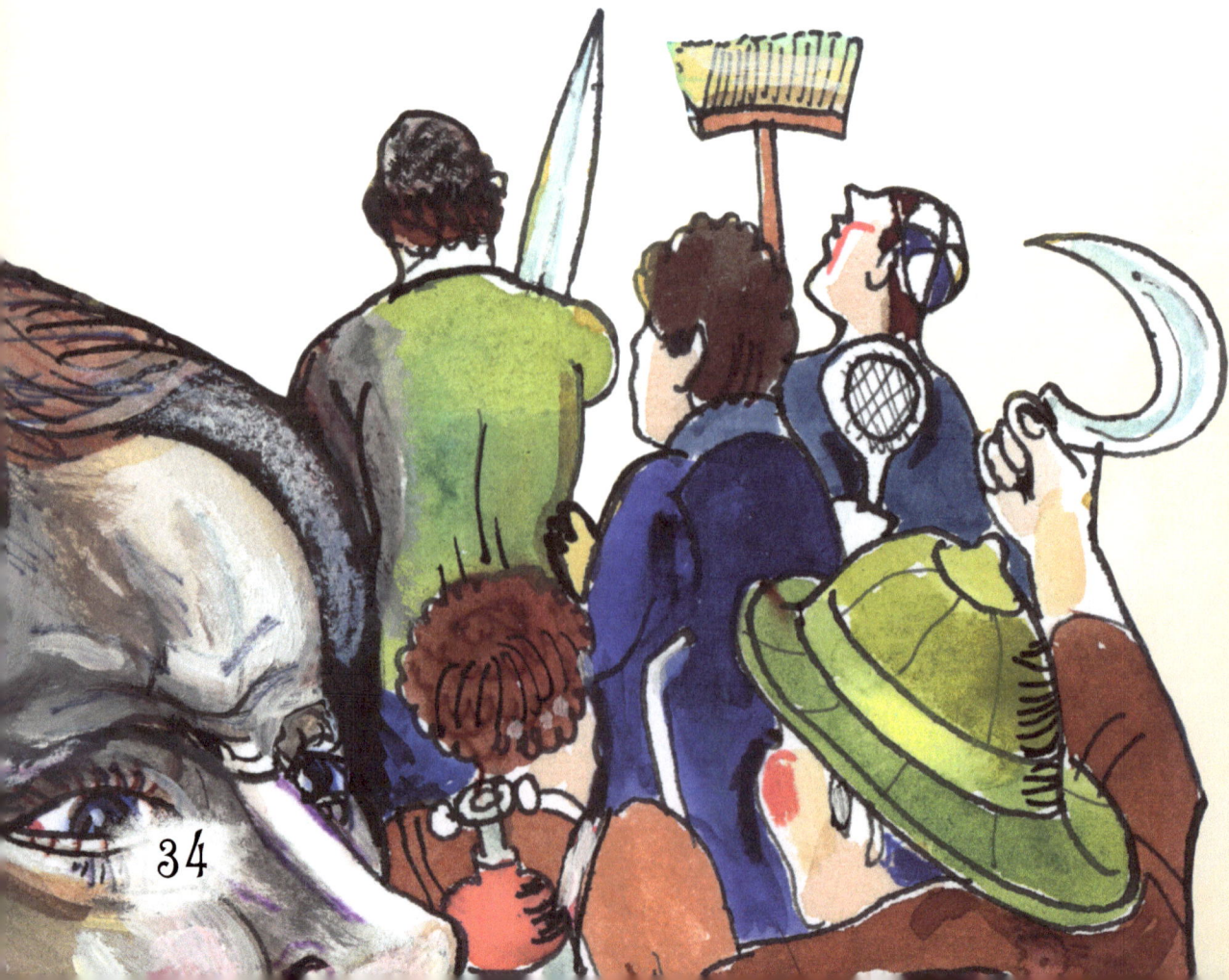

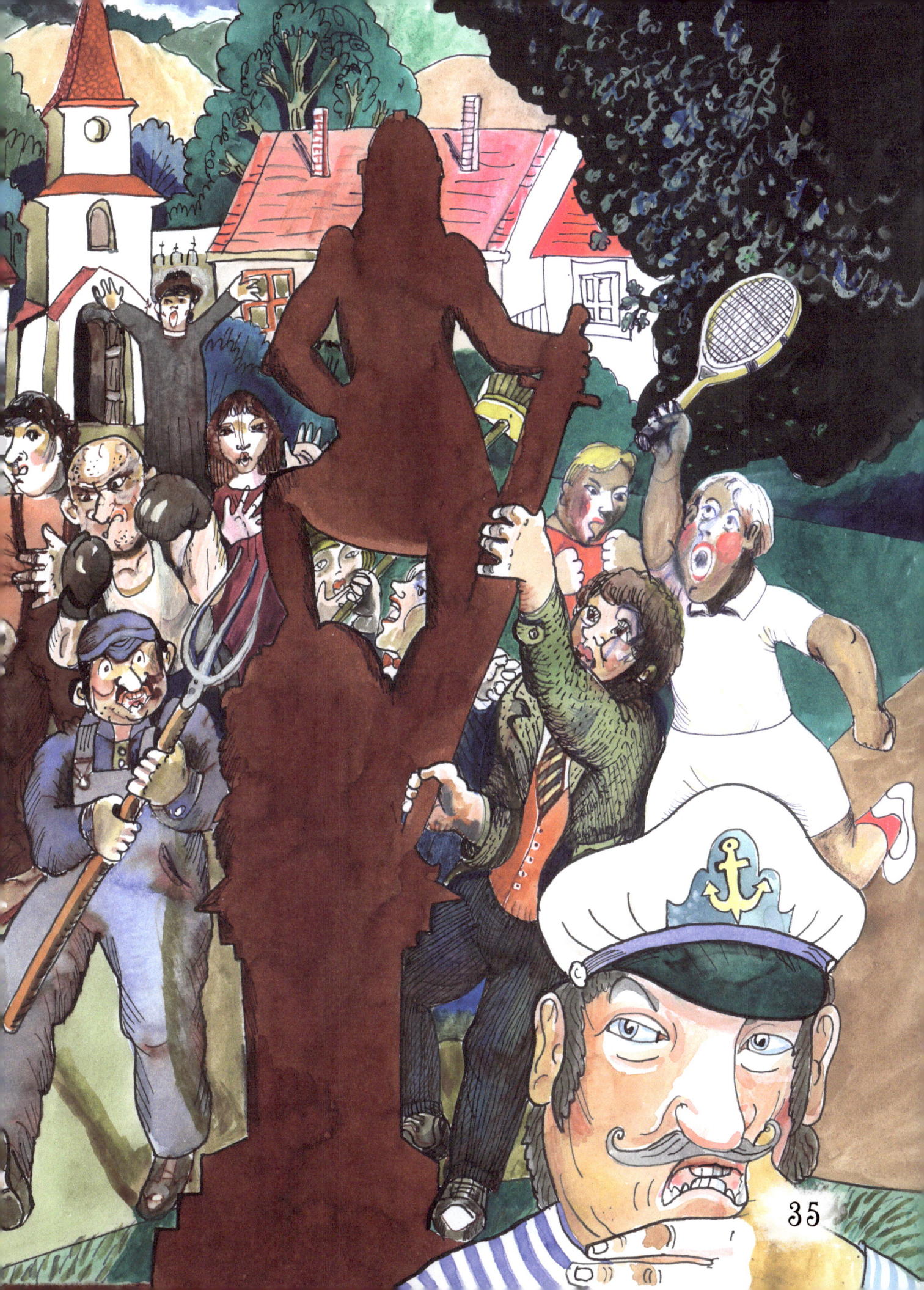

As she stood with one toe on the bridge, Ego the Ogre was rising up from the mucky-yucky mud under the bridge to come and eat her. He crawled slowly out from under the long, long bridge with the mud sucking and slurping at his hands and knees.

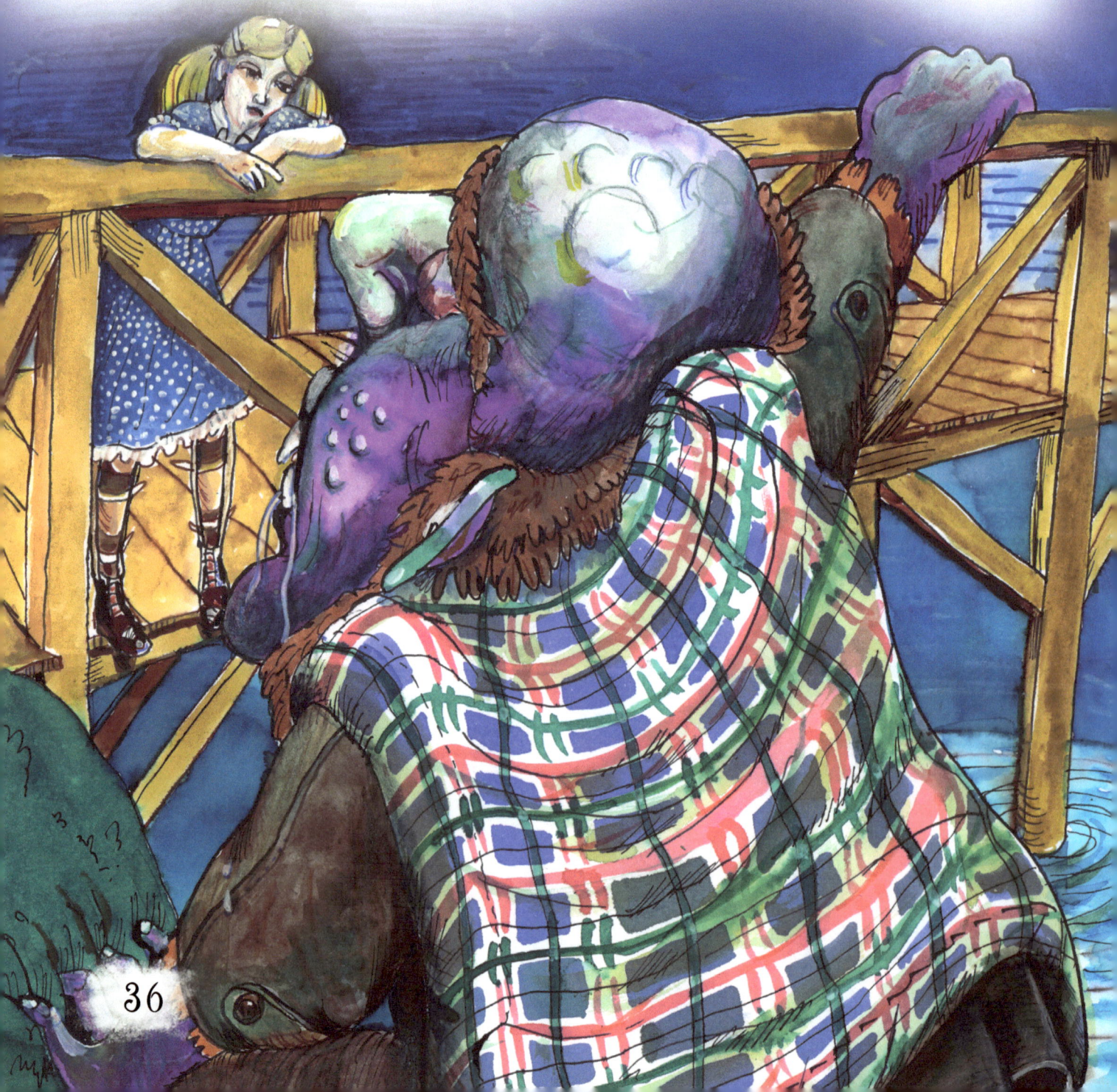

Then he shuffled and snuffled sideways,
as ogres always do, right up to
the tiny little girl. Ego
inflated himself like
a great green goblin
oozing purple
slime.

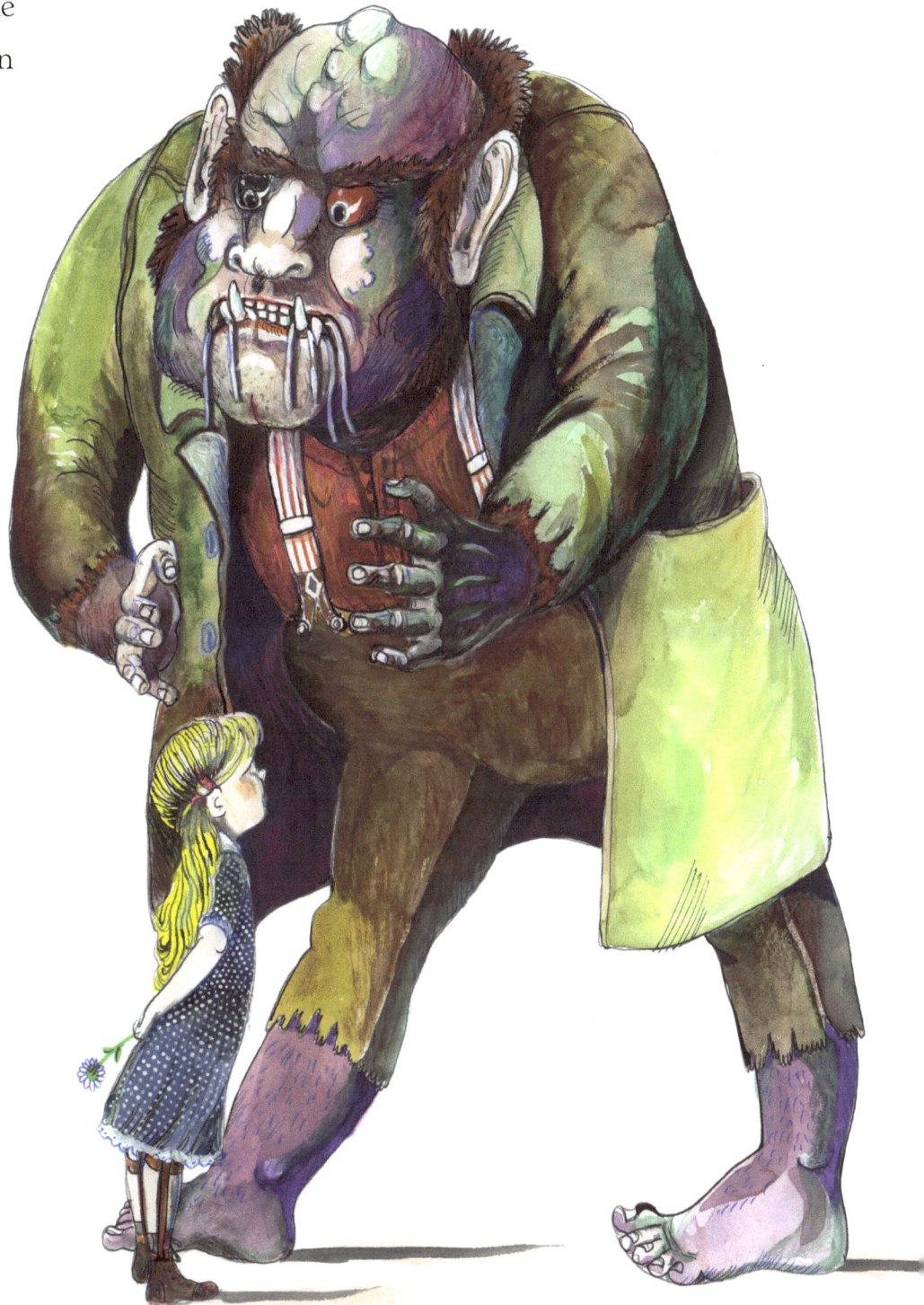

37

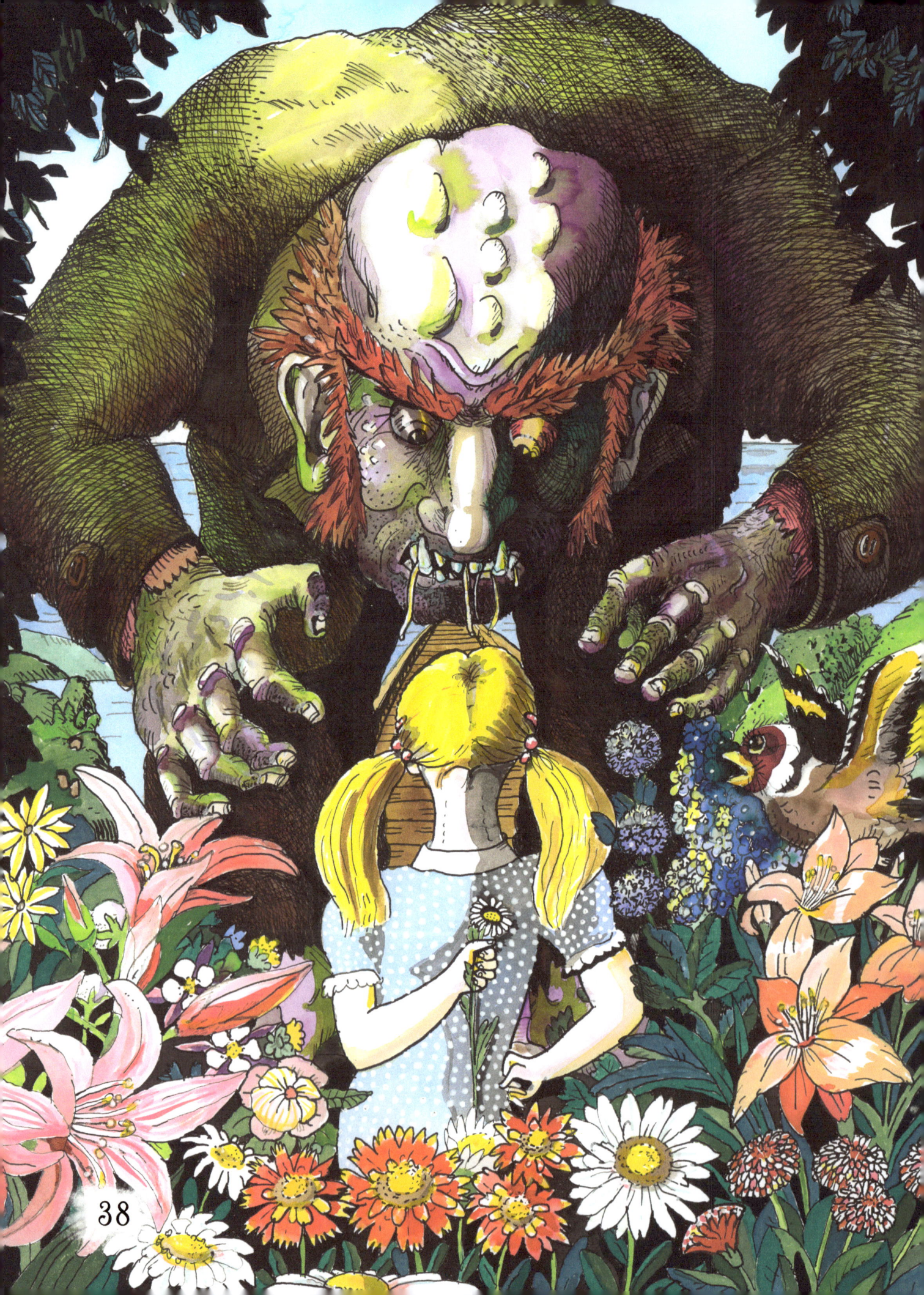

From his teeth, which looked like broken green glass, long strands of smelly old spaghetti dangled over his lips and down his chin just inches from Martina's tiny little upturned face. Ego bellowed,

— "I'm going to eat you up!"

Sweet Little Martina started to get frightened as she stared at that scary old ogre, but she was already in her Happy Place, so she was only afraid for the blink of an eye… and then the fear was gone.

She stood there with her hands behind her back and said nothing at all.

She knew it was wise to wait for someone who is angry to stop yelling before speaking.

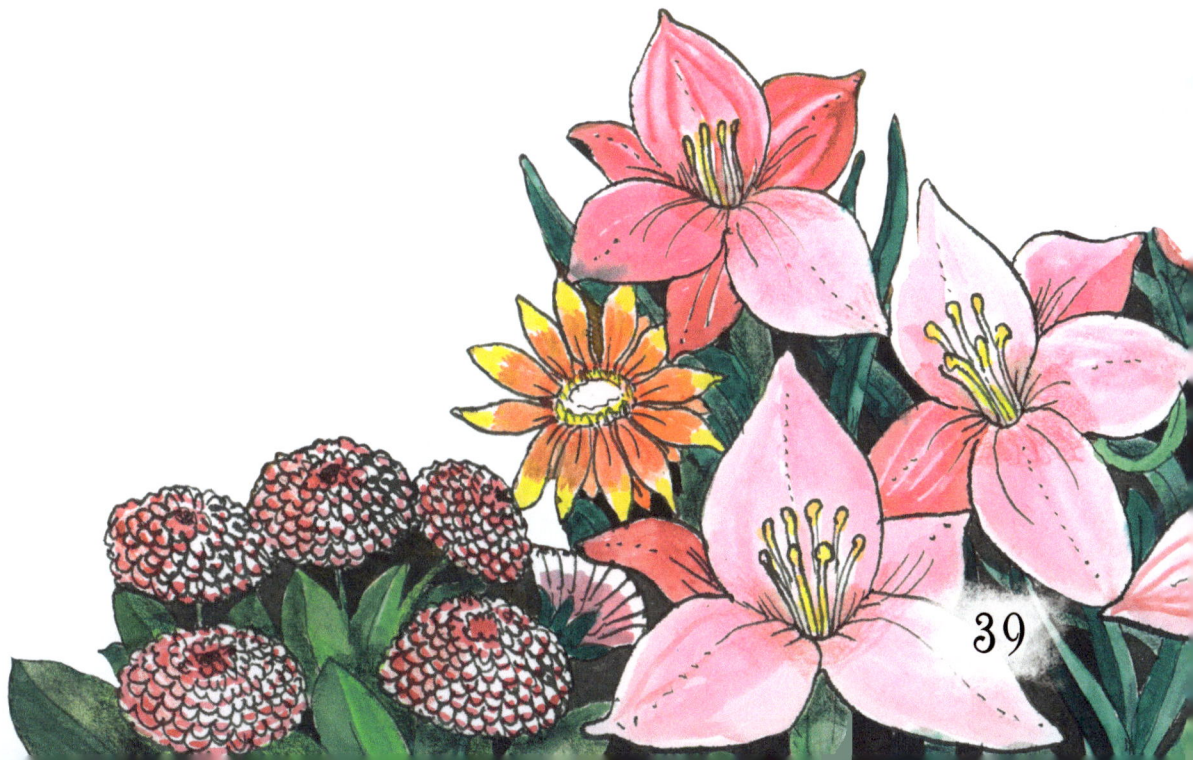

But the angry old ogre roared even louder: "Run away now or I will eat you this very moment!"

Then in her teeny-tiny voice, Sweet Little Martina asked a question that stopped Ego the Ogre in his tracks.

— "Why?" she asked.

— "Why?" he growled, his awful bad breath wrinkling Sweet Little Martina's nose.

— "Why? What do you mean, 'why'?"

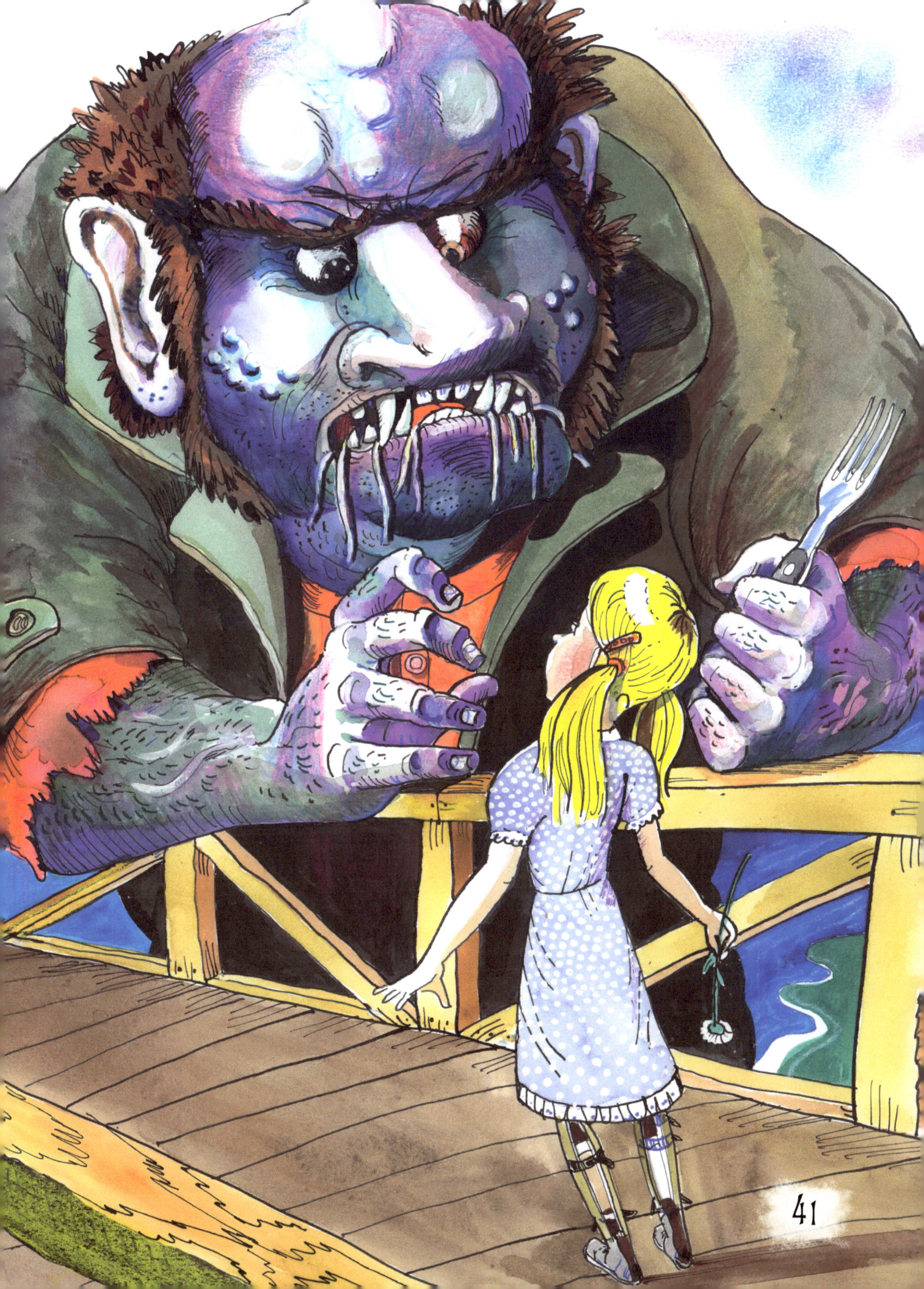

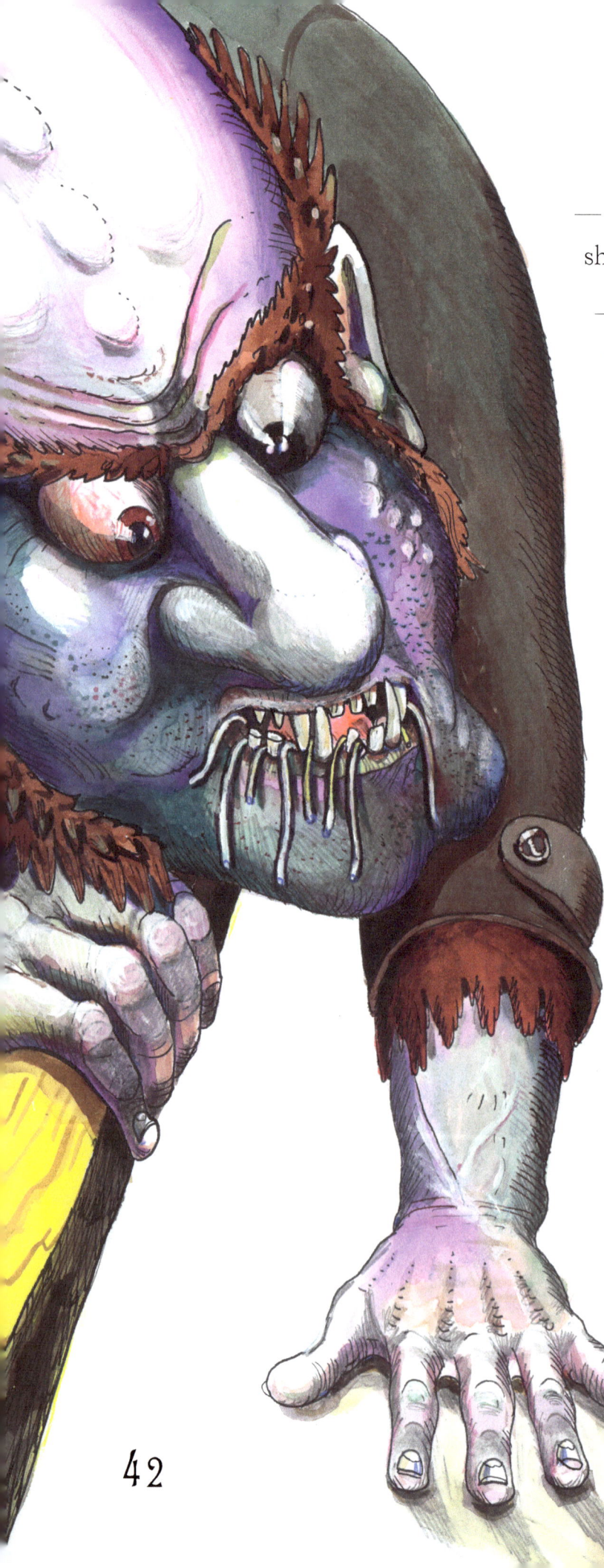

— "Why do you want to eat me?"
she asked quietly.

— "Because, because, uh—I
want to eat you because …"

But he couldn't finish the
sentence.

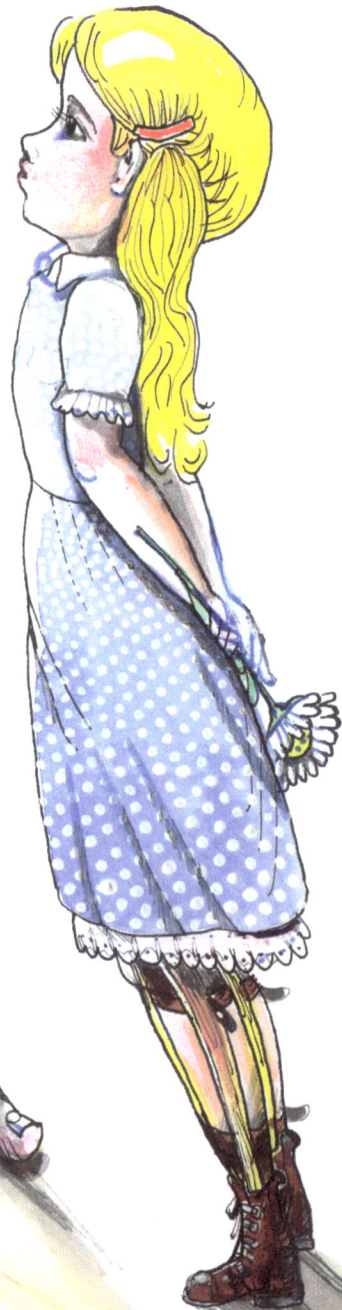

His mind just couldn't think of an answer. In fact, he couldn't think at all. This was most unusual, for Ego the Ogre always had thoughts. He had thoughts about eating little girls. He had thoughts about throwing mud on clean white sheets and stomping on butterflies and eating with his mouth open. He had all kinds of thoughts, but now his mind was completely still. And you know what? It felt good. Ego the Ogre stuttered, a little flustered,

— "I, uh—I can't think of it right now, but I know I have a good reason tucked away in my memory. I … I just know I do."

But he didn't feel as confident as he had a few moments ago. Then Sweet Little Martina asked him something that made his insides feel like jelly. In her teeny-tiny voice, she asked,

— "What do you want most of all?"

It was a simple enough question, but somehow, no matter what Ego the Ogre tried to say in reply, it didn't seem quite right. Did he want a treasure fit for a king? No. Did he want to eat Sweet Little Martina? Not really. He kind of liked this pale little girl. Did he want more food? A clean new bridge to live under? Or even a red toy fire engine that could go really, really fast? No, no, no! When he thought about it, he really didn't know what he wanted most of all. Maybe he wanted Nothing.

Ego the Ogre looked down upon Sweet Little Martina's innocent face, and he felt confused because he really didn't want to hurt anyone or anything.

As he gazed at her, Sweet Little Martina brought her hands from behind her back and handed Ego the Ogre the single sunshine daisy she had picked from the meadow by the side of the road.

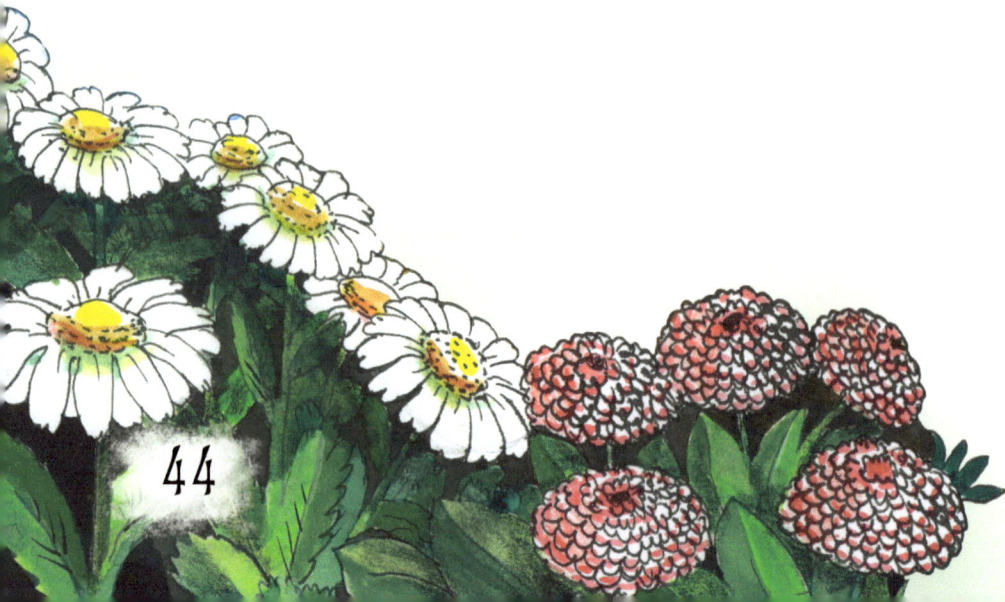

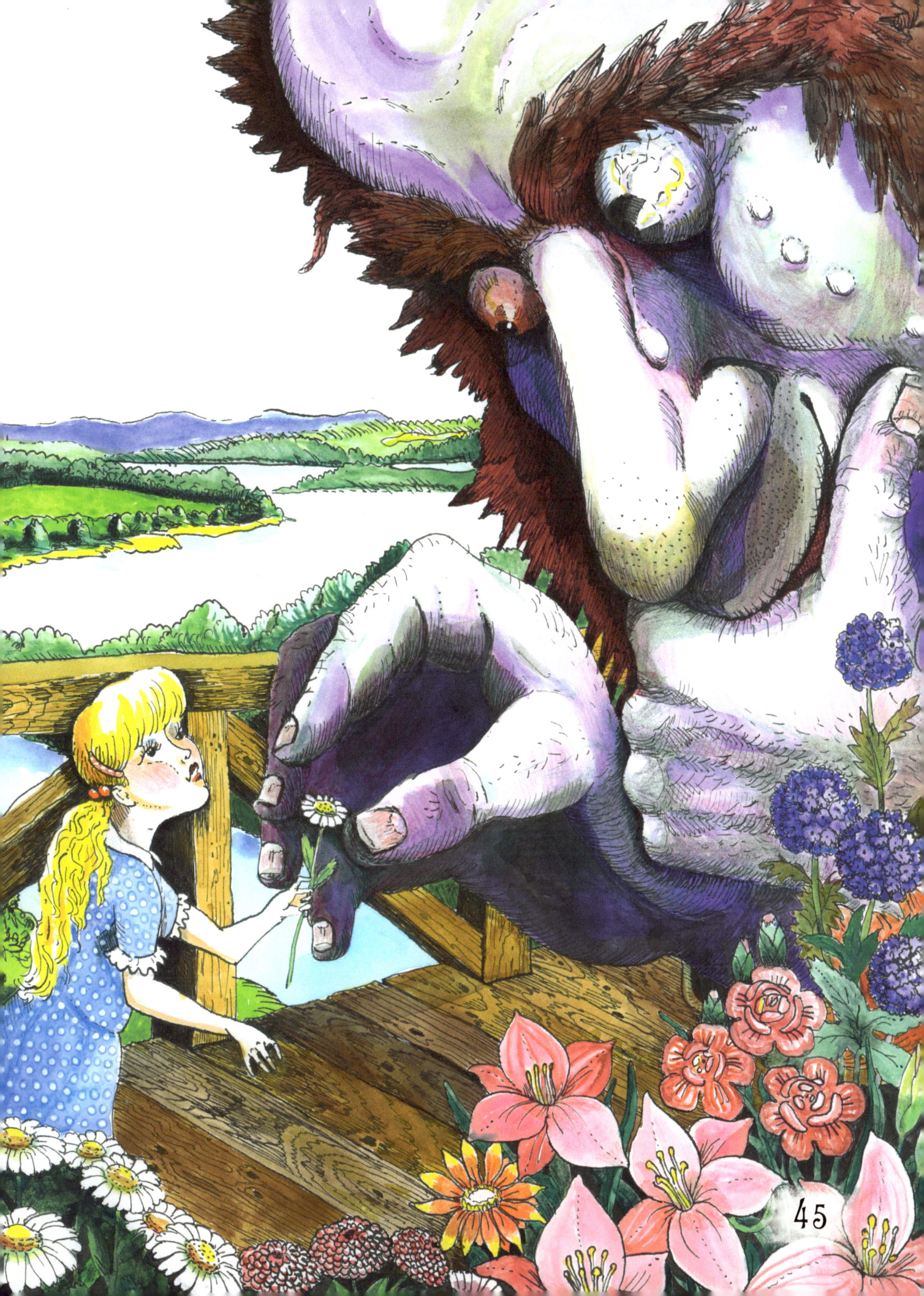

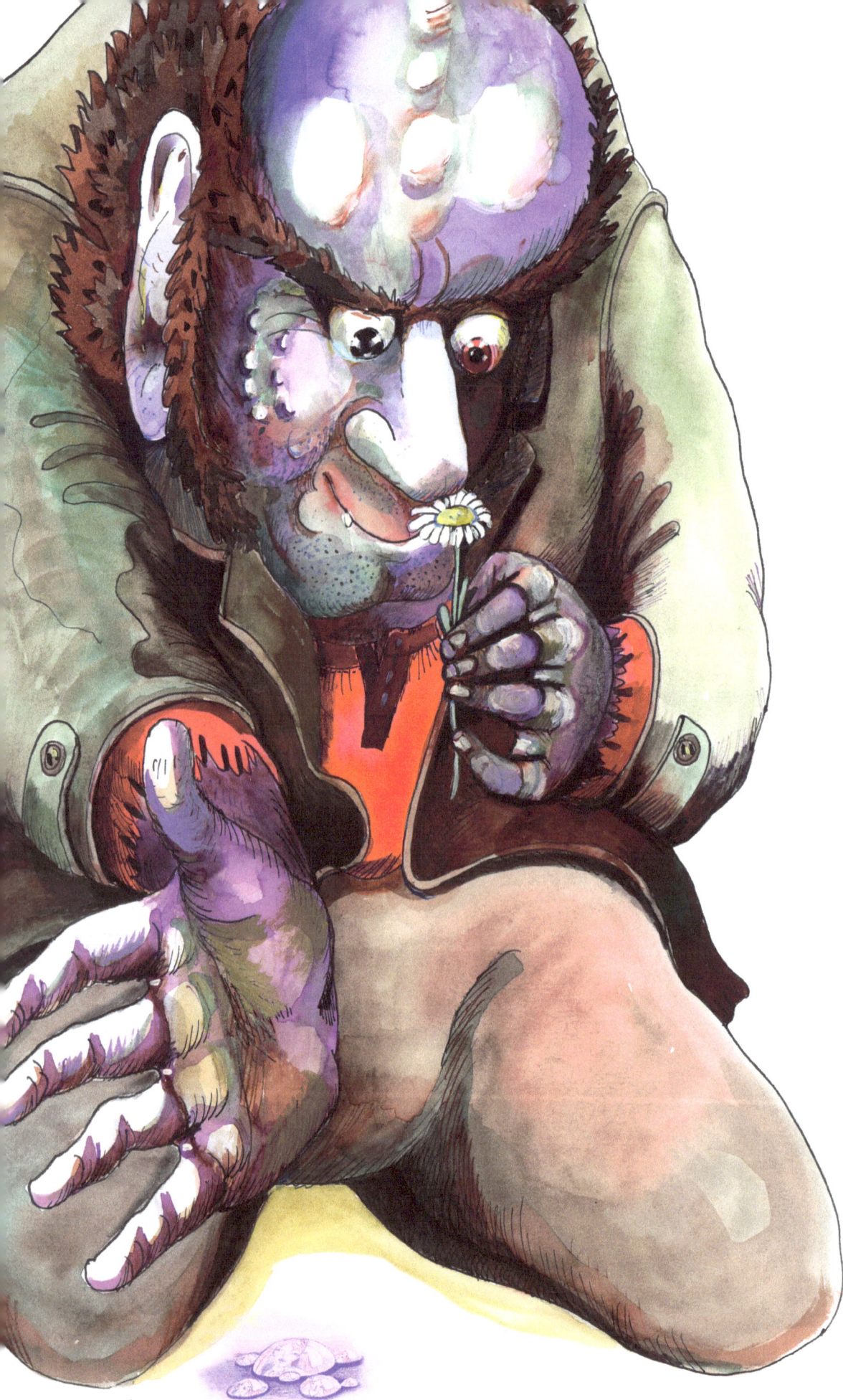

A giant green glistening tear formed in the ogre's black eye, rolled off his pointed cheek, and fell to the ground, making a crater in the dust. Sweet Little Martina said,

— "Don't cry, Mr. Ogre. I will teach you how to find the Happy Place inside you, and you will never be sad again."

And she did.

The ogre felt his heart getting bigger and bigger like a balloon filled with helium. It felt like it was going to fill his whole chest so that he could float all the way up beyond the clouds. He was really, really happy for the first time in his life; and he was very thankful to Sweet Little Martina for showing him to his Happy Place.

Then Ego bowed deeply and swept his huge green arm toward the long, long bridge. And then he spoke in a gentle voice that made Sweet Little Martina feel even happier than before.

He said softly, "You may pass."

And she did.

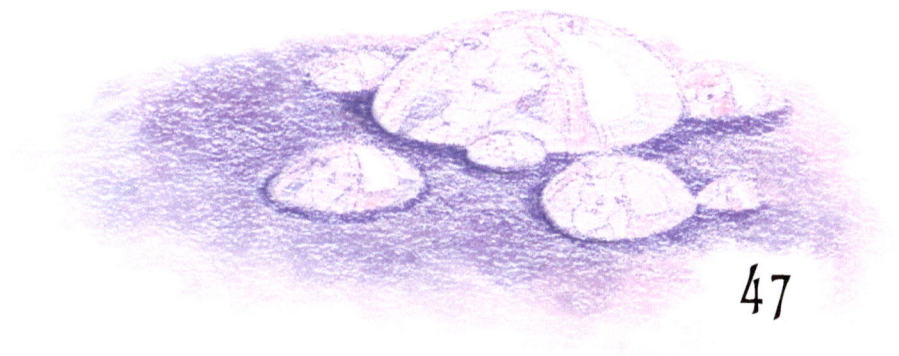

Meanwhile, the townspeople were moving slowly along the road to the long, long bridge to save Sweet Little Martina from the evil old ogre. They didn't know that she was already crossing to the other side of the beautiful blue lake. They were moving slowly because the ones in the front of the line kept finding excuses to go to the back of the line.

Twenty-three townsfolk had to stop and tie their shoes while the rest of the villagers walked past. Fourteen got rocks in their shoes or complained of blisters and had to sit down, and seven had sudden attacks of lumbago. Eleven remembered that they'd left the burners burning on their stoves back in the busy little village.

Most of them had never cooked a day in their lives, but promised themselves that they would start cooking that very day as long as they did not have to come face-to-face with mean old Ego the Ogre.

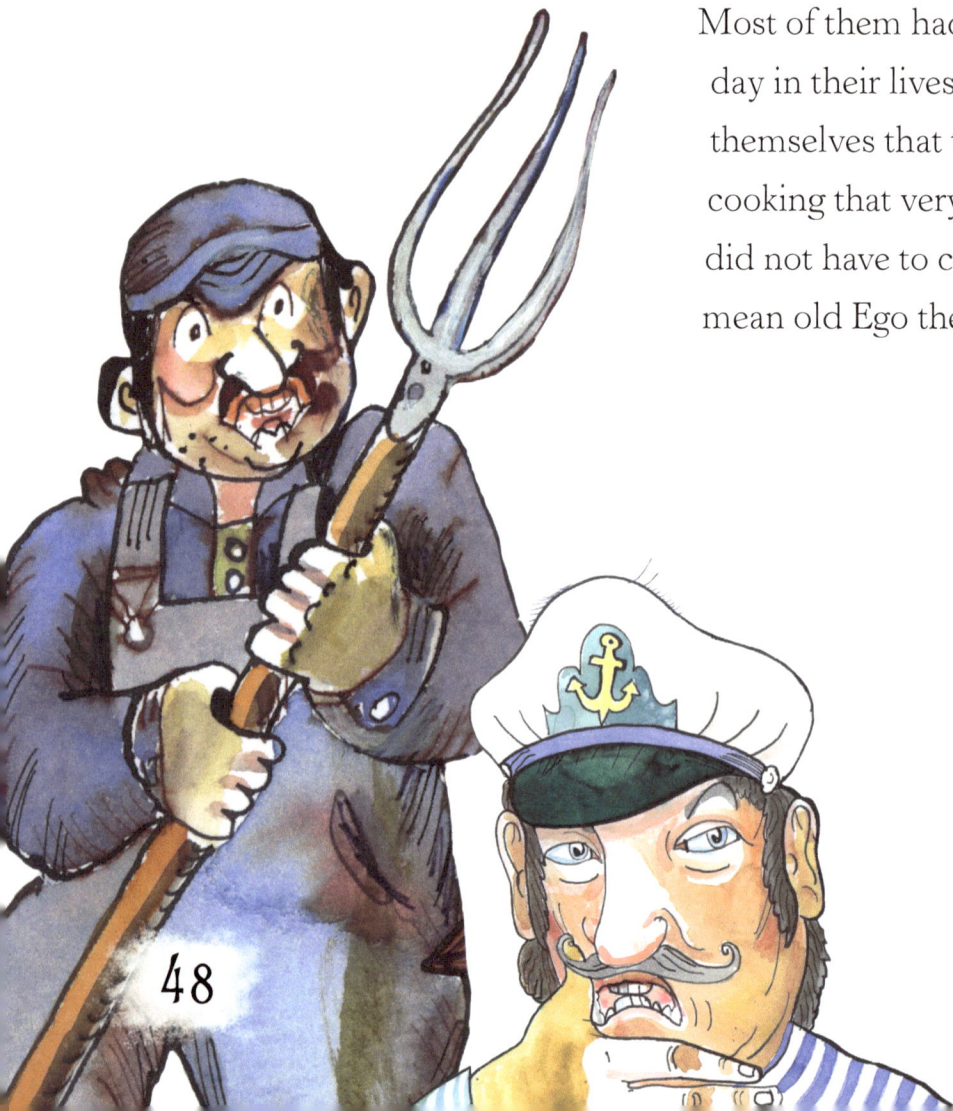

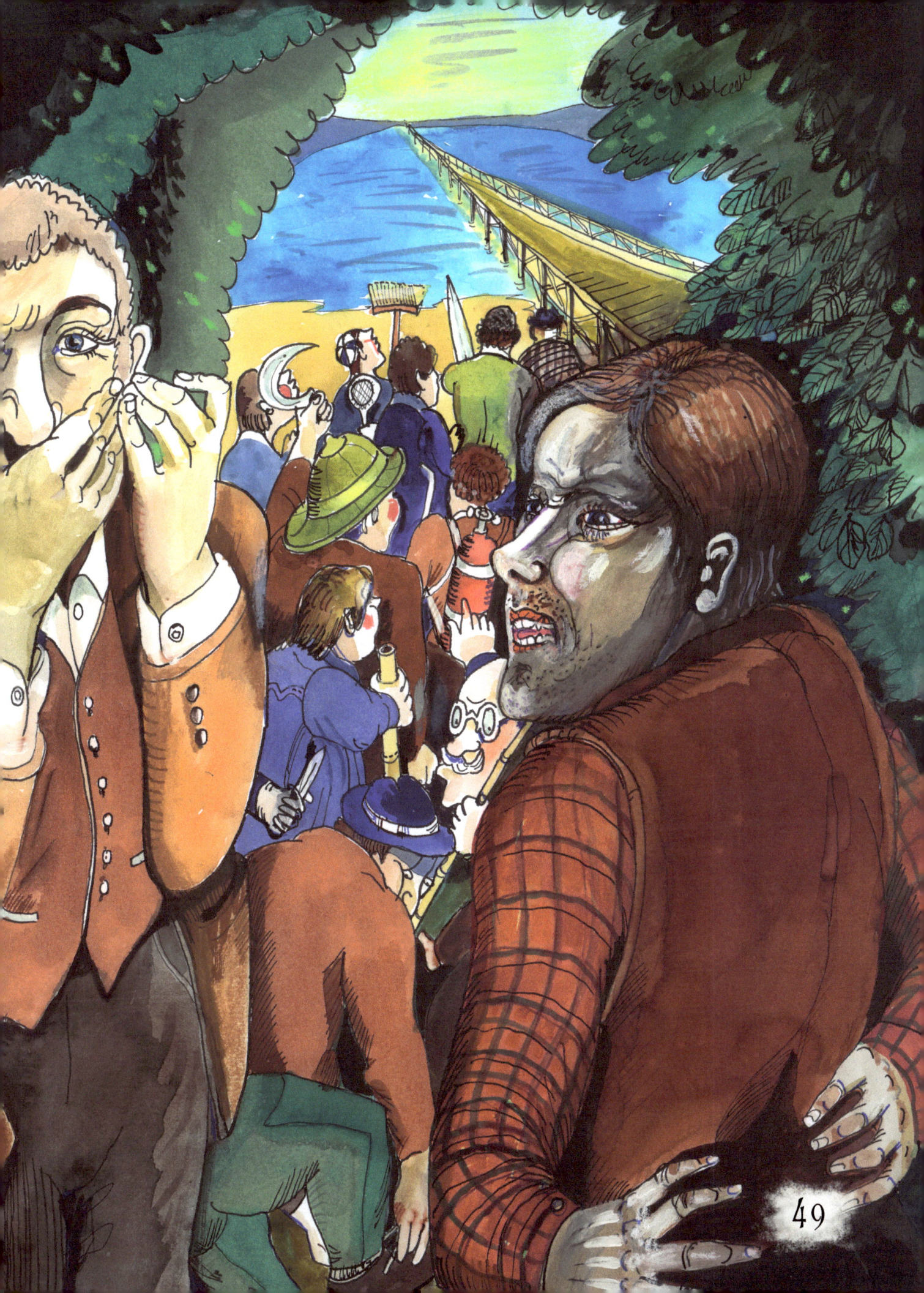

Finally, the remaining villagers arrived at the long, long bridge over the beautiful blue lake. They saw Ego the Ogre standing at the entrance of the bridge smelling a daisy. They knew right away that it must be Sweet Little Martina's daisy, because no self-respecting ogre would ever sniff a dainty daisy. Everyone was very upset and very afraid, and one person yelled out,

— "What have you done with our Sweet Little Martina?"
Ego the Ogre replied,

— "I let her go over the long, long bridge."

— "Liar!" yelled another villager. "You've eaten her!" And all the others joined in, yelling and screaming and shaking their brooms and tennis rackets at the surprised ogre.

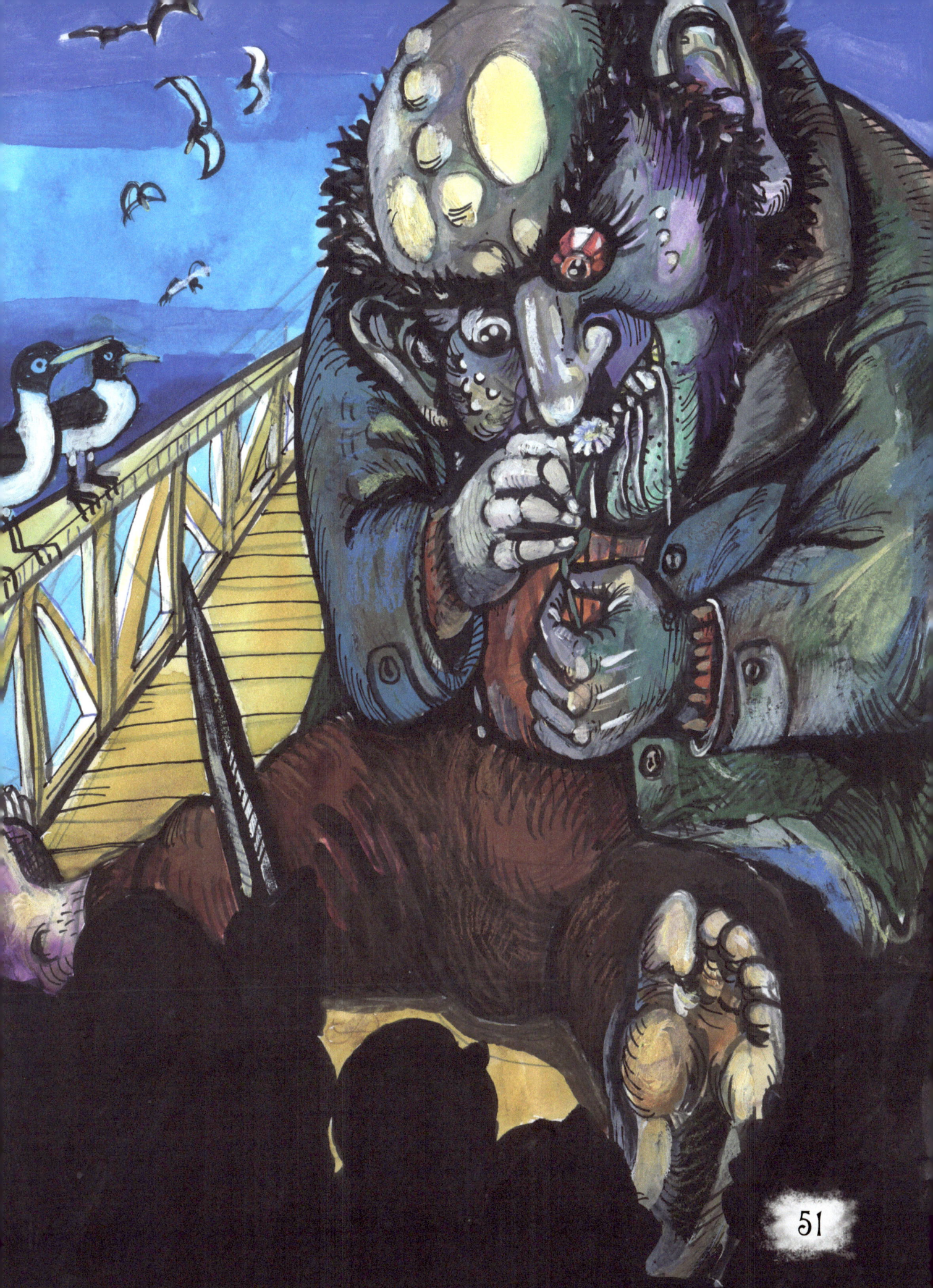

— "It's true," Ego replied.

— "She went over to the other side of the beautiful blue lake."

The villagers became more enraged than they were afraid, and pressed in toward Ego the Ogre. The man with the wobbly old sword stayed right behind the people in front. He thought that while Ego the Ogre was busy eating the people in front, he would have time to run away. Even though he had the wobbly old sword, he wasn't very brave. He only wanted people to think so.

Just then Ego the Ogre stepped forward to show the townspeople the daisy and tell them that Sweet Little Martina gave it to him. He

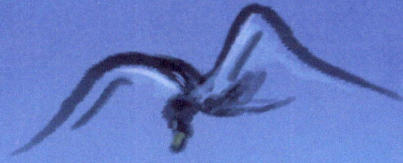

wanted to tell them that she showed him where his Happy Place was and that she was now his friend.

She had even cleared his mind of bad, bad thoughts; and now he felt a funny feeling inside that made him happy and want to help people instead of hurt them.

When he stepped toward the villagers to show them the daisy, however, the people in the front of the line fell backward and the people behind the man with the wobbly old sword pushed him forward at the same time.

The man with the wobbly old sword stumbled and fell forward, and the sword stabbed Ego the Ogre in the right kneecap.

Now, if you or I were stabbed in the right kneecap with a wobbly old sword, it might hurt a lot, but we would be just fine after a little clean water, a bandage, and some love. But this is not so for ogres. The right kneecap is the only place that you can hurt an ogre. And a stab from a wobbly old sword is the only thing that can kill an ogre.

As the villagers watched, they saw the ogre fall down holding his right knee, and then a very strange thing happened.

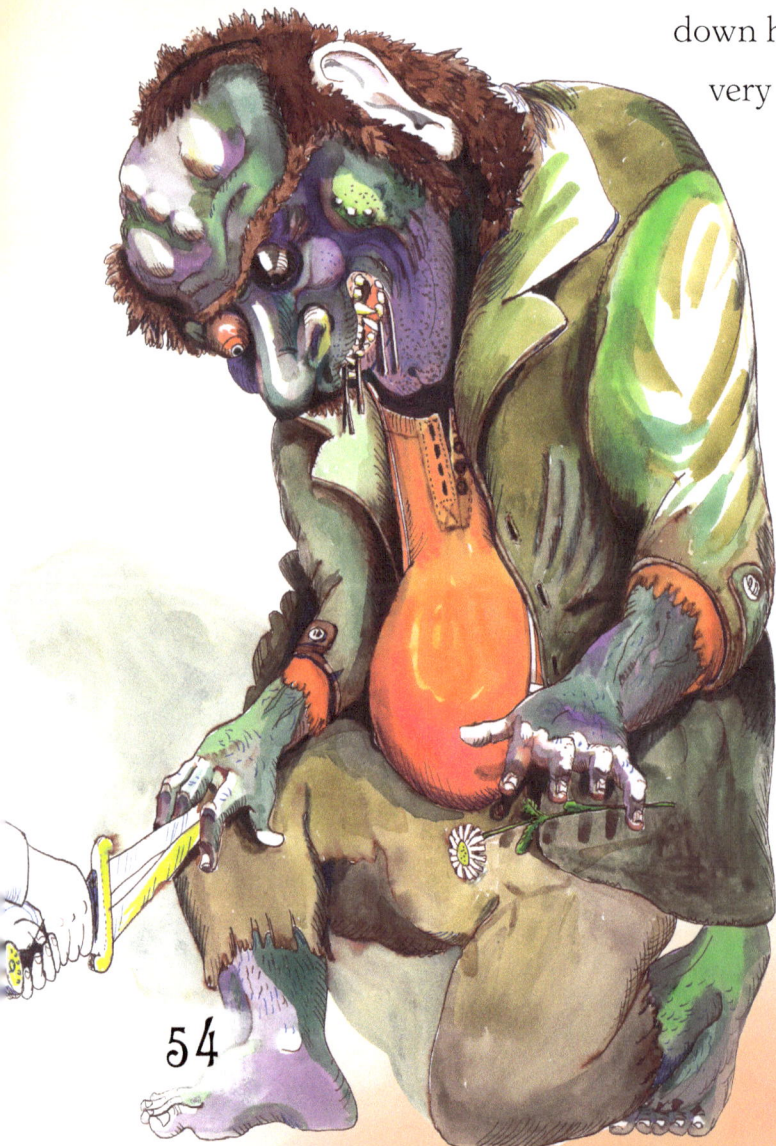

Ego the Ogre's body started to get lighter and lighter, as if it were turning into angel dust. Next it turned into light and disappeared into thin air.

One moment he was there, and the next—poof—he was gone.

When he got stabbed in the right kneecap, Ego felt a strange sensation. It was as if his heart really was expanding and he really did begin to float up, up, up beyond the clouds. As he was floating up beyond the clouds, Ego was looking down and saw the man who had stabbed him raise his wobbly old sword in the air and yell,

— "I did it! I killed the mean old ogre with my skill and cunning. I am the bravest man in the village, and you should all buy me stuff and be nice to me forever and ever."

Right then, another strange thing happened, but the villagers were getting used to strange things happening by now because this had been a day full of strange events … and it wasn't even lunchtime yet. What they saw happening to the man with the sword made them step back and say,

— "Oh my!"

The man with the wobbly old sword who was bragging about bravely killing the mean old ogre was changing. His skin was growing purple with green spots, and it was becoming slimy and smelly and bumpy. He grew jagged teeth like broken green glass with strings of old spaghetti hanging down. His breath began to smell like tuna fish and broccoli and dirty socks all mixed together. And his eyes changed color: one red and one black. The townspeople began pointing and chanting,

— "Ego the Ogre, Ego the Ogre, Ego the Ogre!"

The wobbly old sword fell from the man's hand, slid down the bank into the clear deep water of the beautiful blue lake, and was never seen again. And the bragging man really did turn into a mean old ogre. He was so ashamed that he slunk down the bank to hide under the long, long bridge. Later that night, he stole away to live in a cave deep in the Long-way-away Mountains and was never seen again.

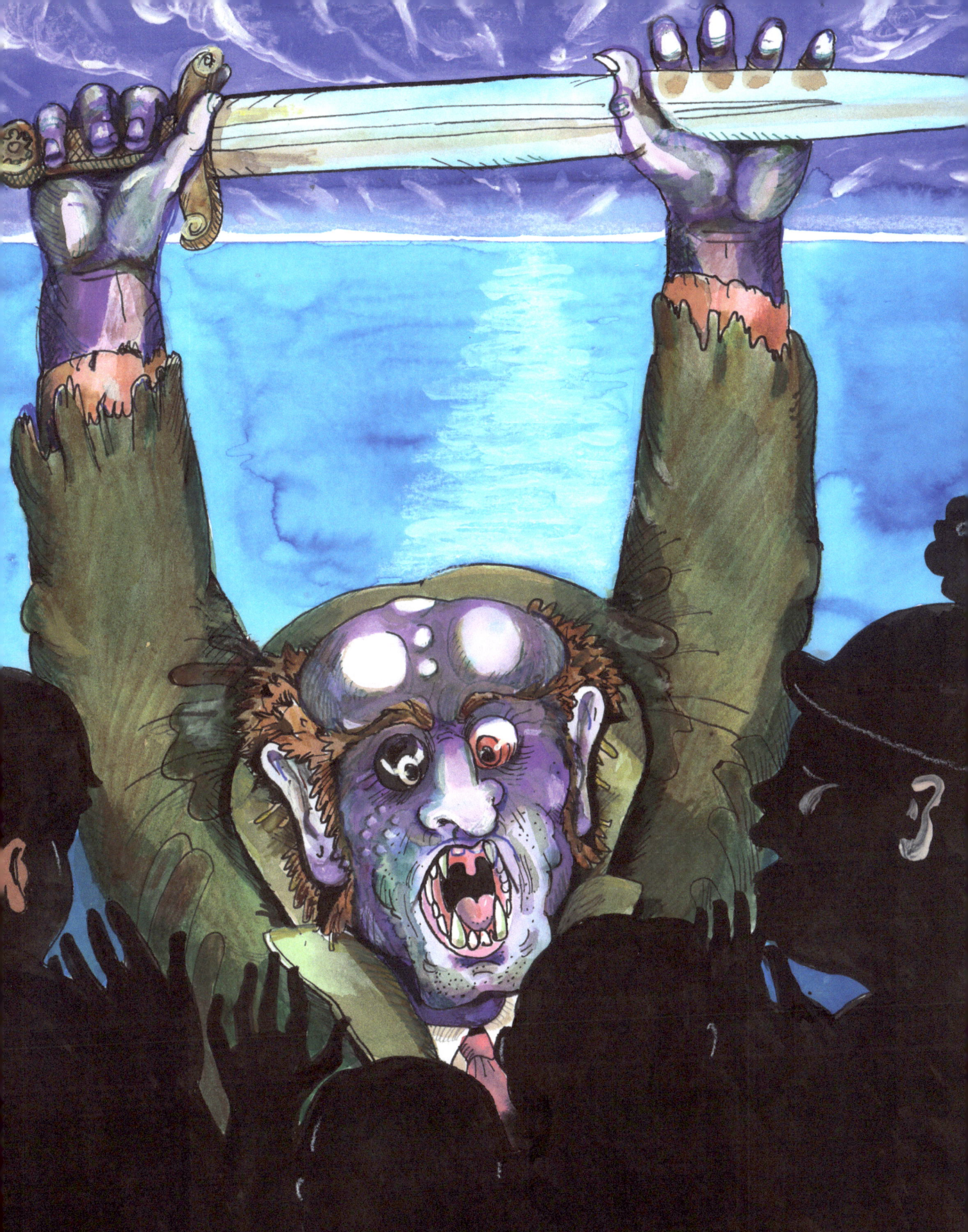

Then another strange thing happened. (Okay, okay … this is the last strange thing for this story, I promise.)

There, walking back from the other side of the beautiful blue lake, was Sweet Little Martina smiling more sweetly than she had ever smiled before. And guess what? She was walking without braces on her legs! All the villagers ran around her and lifted her up on their shoulders, as her father and mother hugged and kissed her and told her how happy they were that she had come back to them.

— They asked, "Where have you been?"

— And Sweet Little Martina answered, "I'll tell you!"

And this is what she told the villagers about her journey across the long, long bridge:

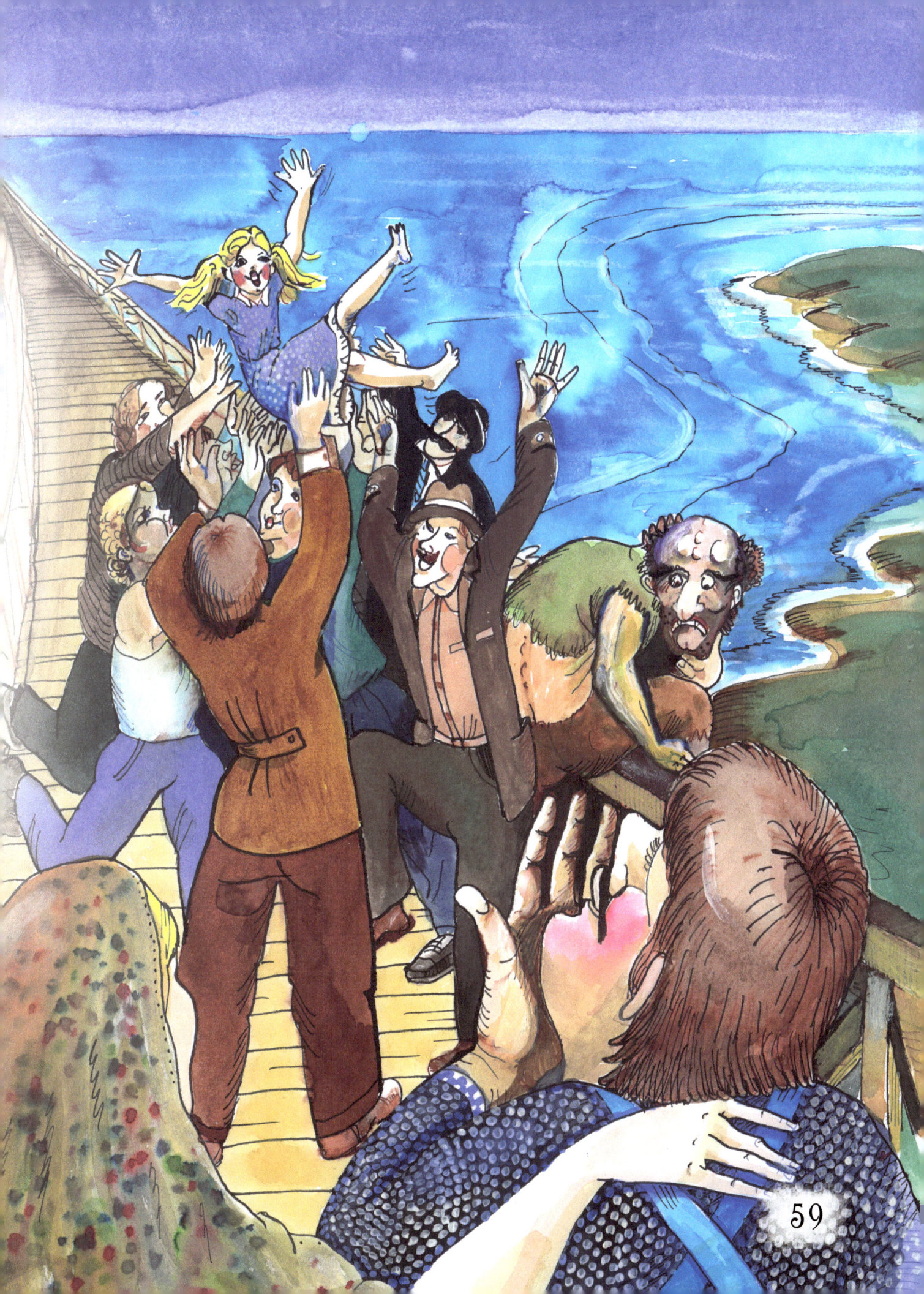

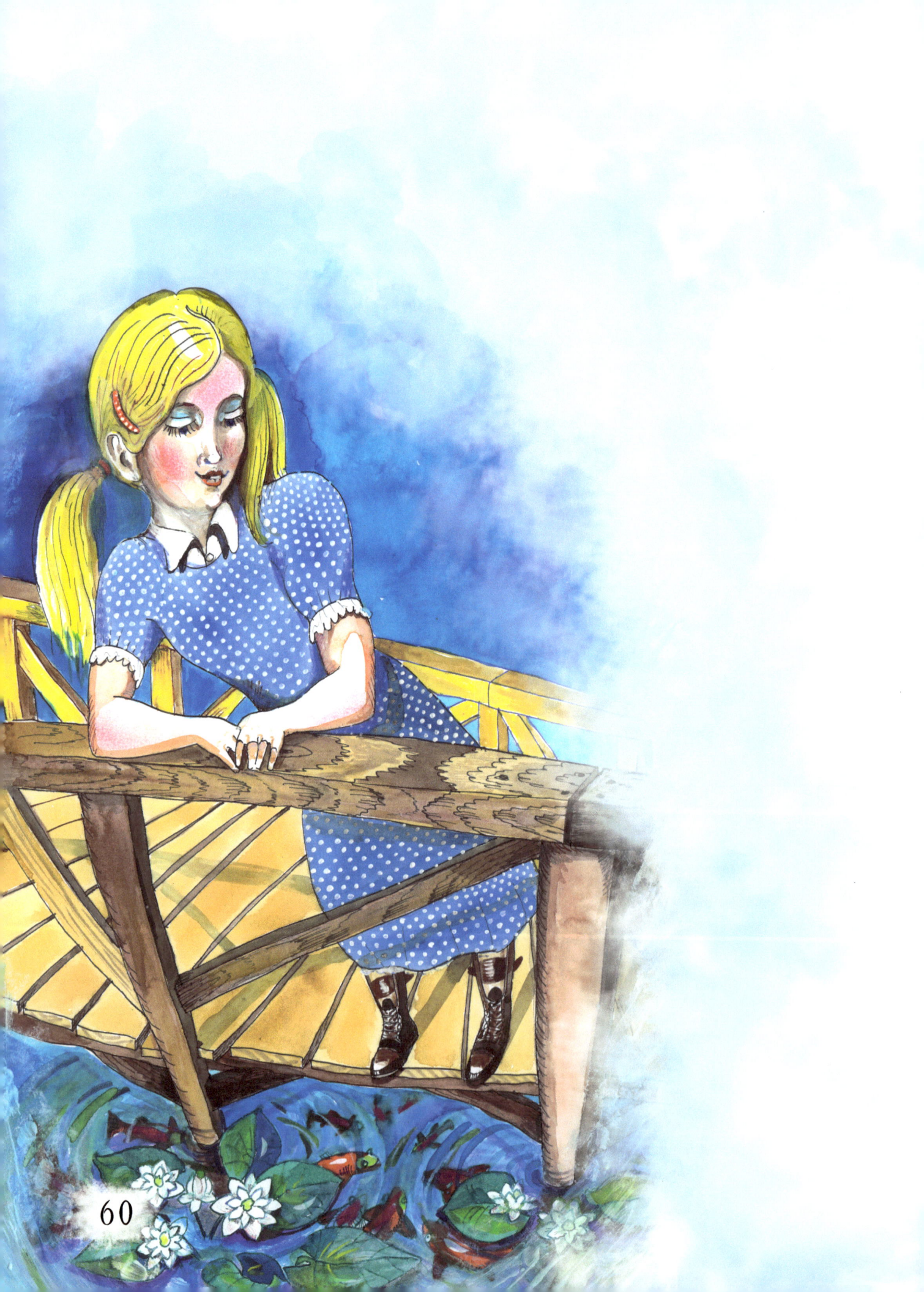

— "I walked a long way and didn't think I would be able to walk all the way to the end of the long, long bridge because my braces made my legs so very tired."

— "I stopped to look into the water of the beautiful blue lake, and I could see shimmering fishes singing and playing among the blossoming lake flowers down below. It was all very beautiful and I wanted to stay, but a little voice in my heart urged me to go on."

— "So I did."

— "I walked and I walked and I walked some more, and then I finally saw the end of the long, long bridge. When I got there, I looked out over the land and there was nothing there."

— "I peered into the nothingness for some time but still could not see anything. Then I stepped off the long, long bridge into the land of Nothing, and I felt my feet get all tingly and begin to dissolve. It wasn't a bad feeling. It was wonderful—like stepping into a warm bath but without getting wet. Then my legs dissolved into nothing and my tummy and chest and arms and head all dissolved into nothing."

— "I don't know how long I was there, but I didn't fall asleep. I was awake, but I didn't see or hear or feel anything. All of a sudden, I found myself standing back on the long, long bridge facing home."

— "I turned and started to walk the long way back home, and then something wonderful happened."

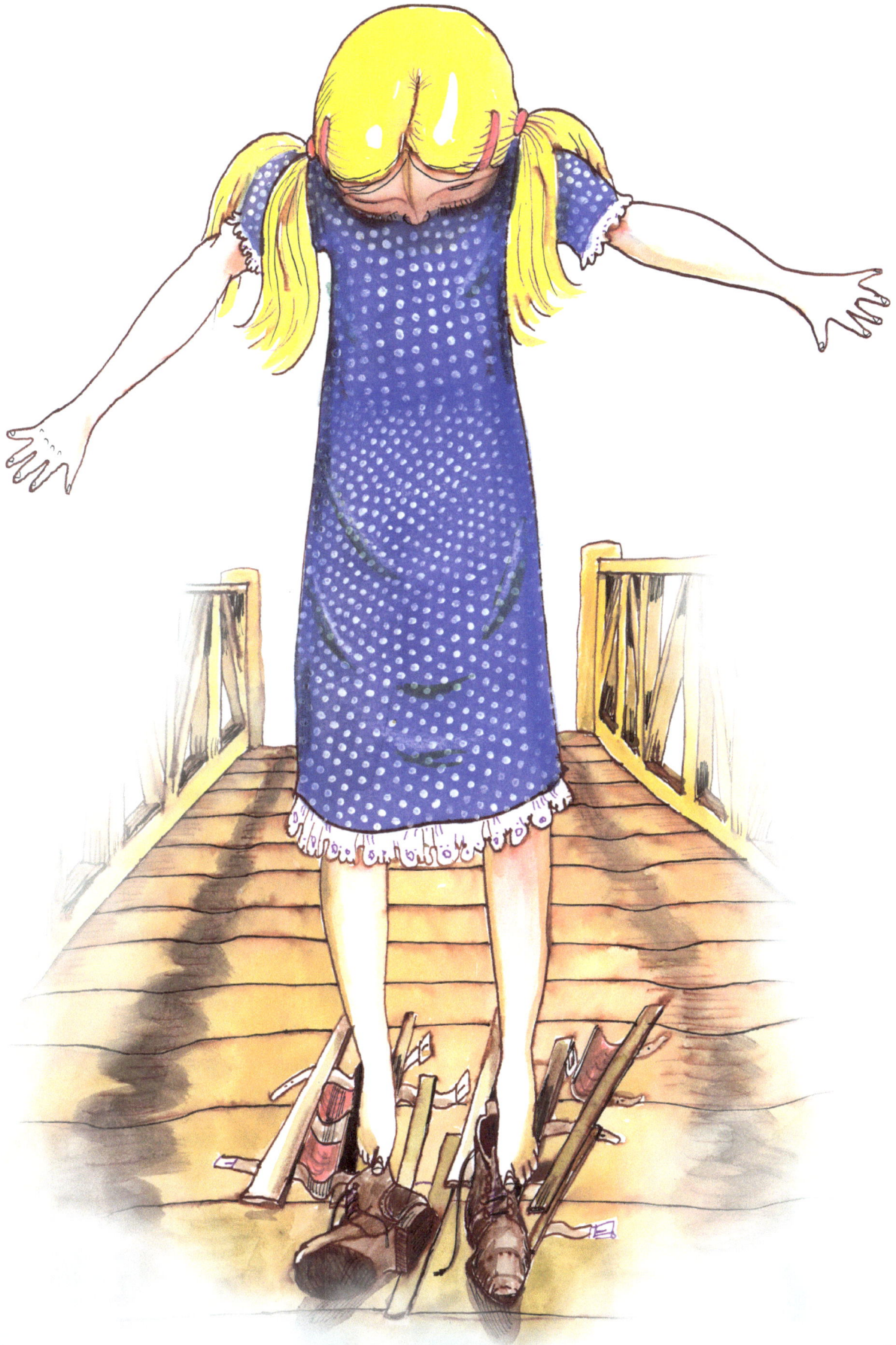

— "My braces fell off my legs; and I floated up, up, and away from the long, long bridge high up into the air."

— "Up, up, up I went like a beautiful bird. I was flying!"

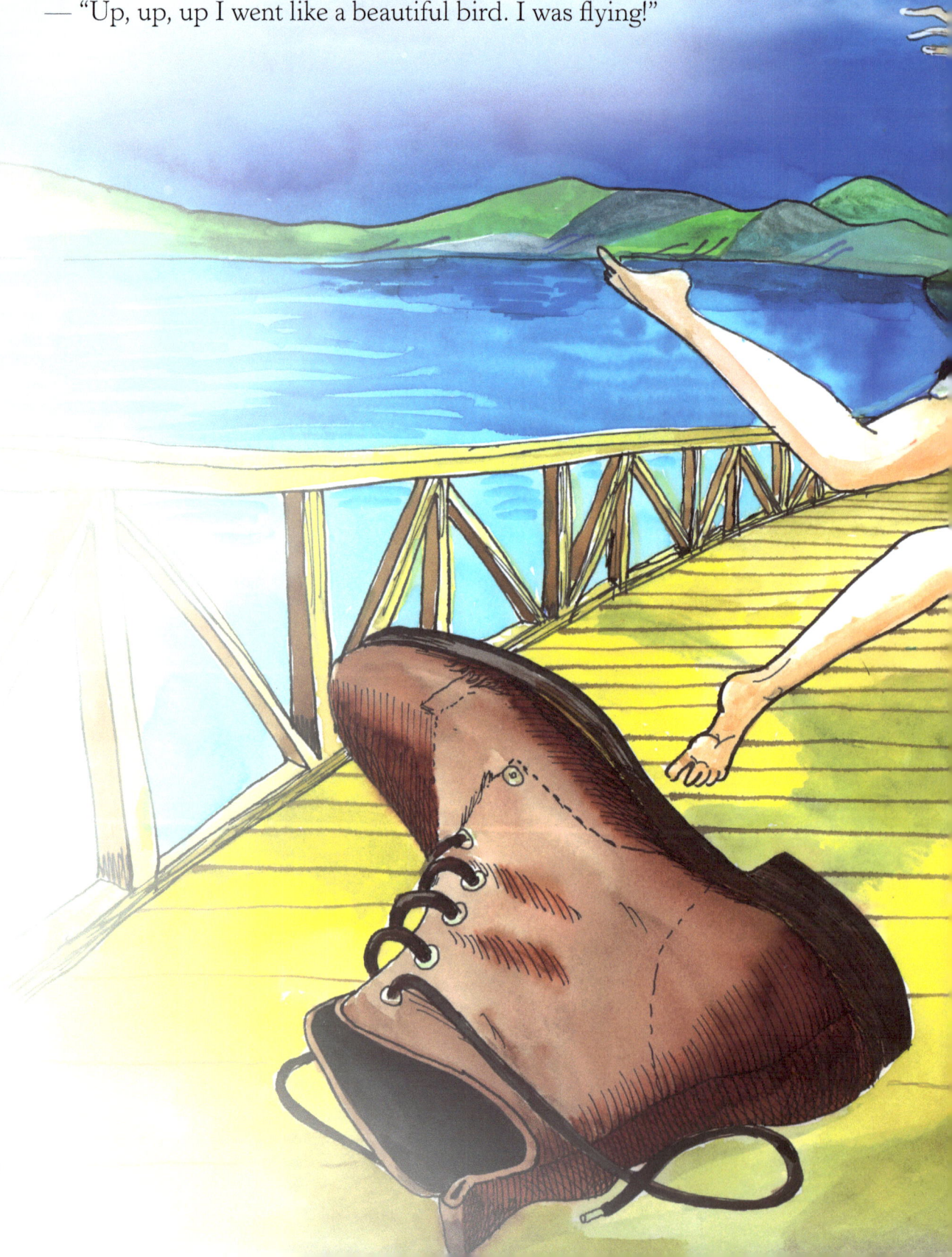

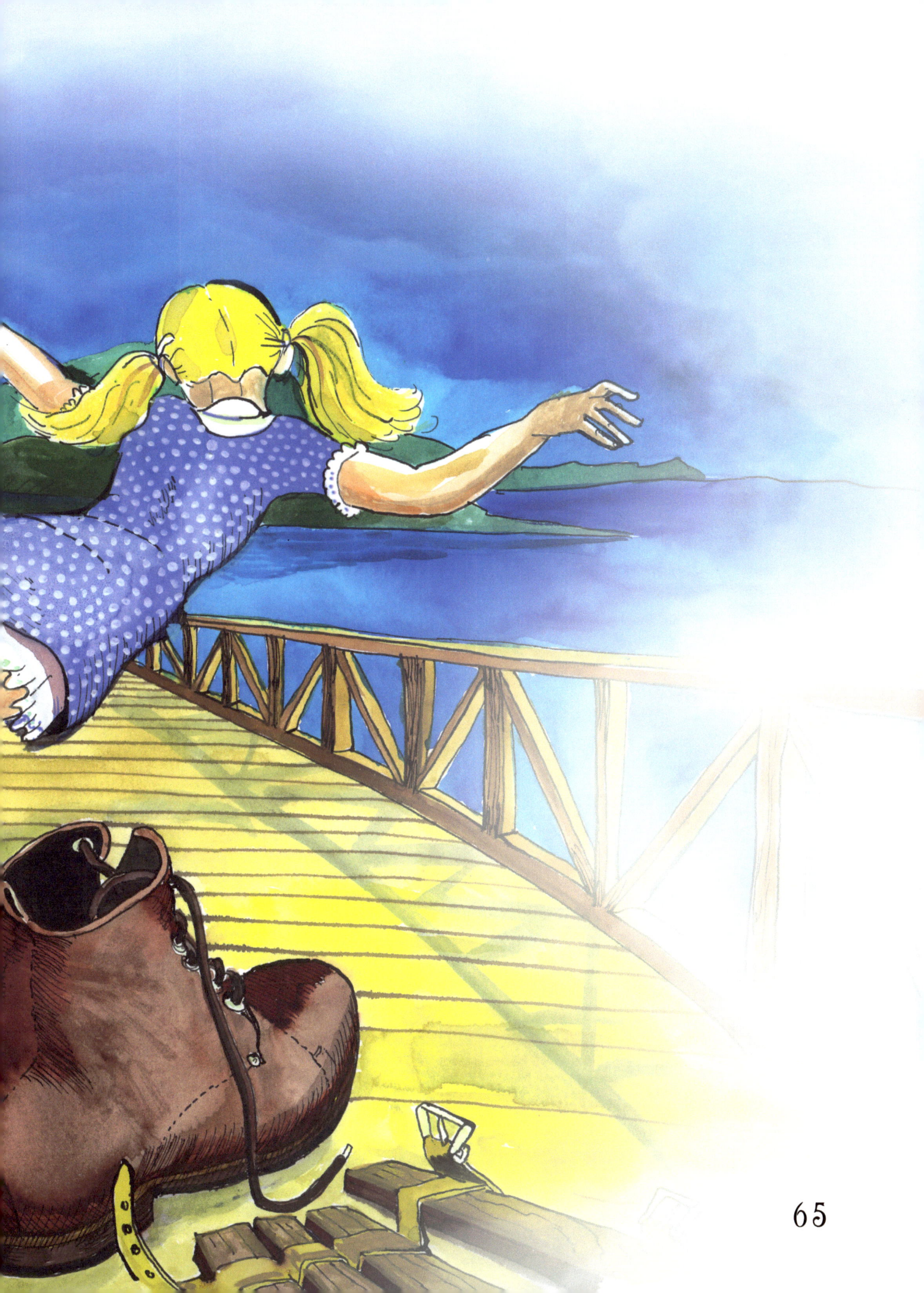

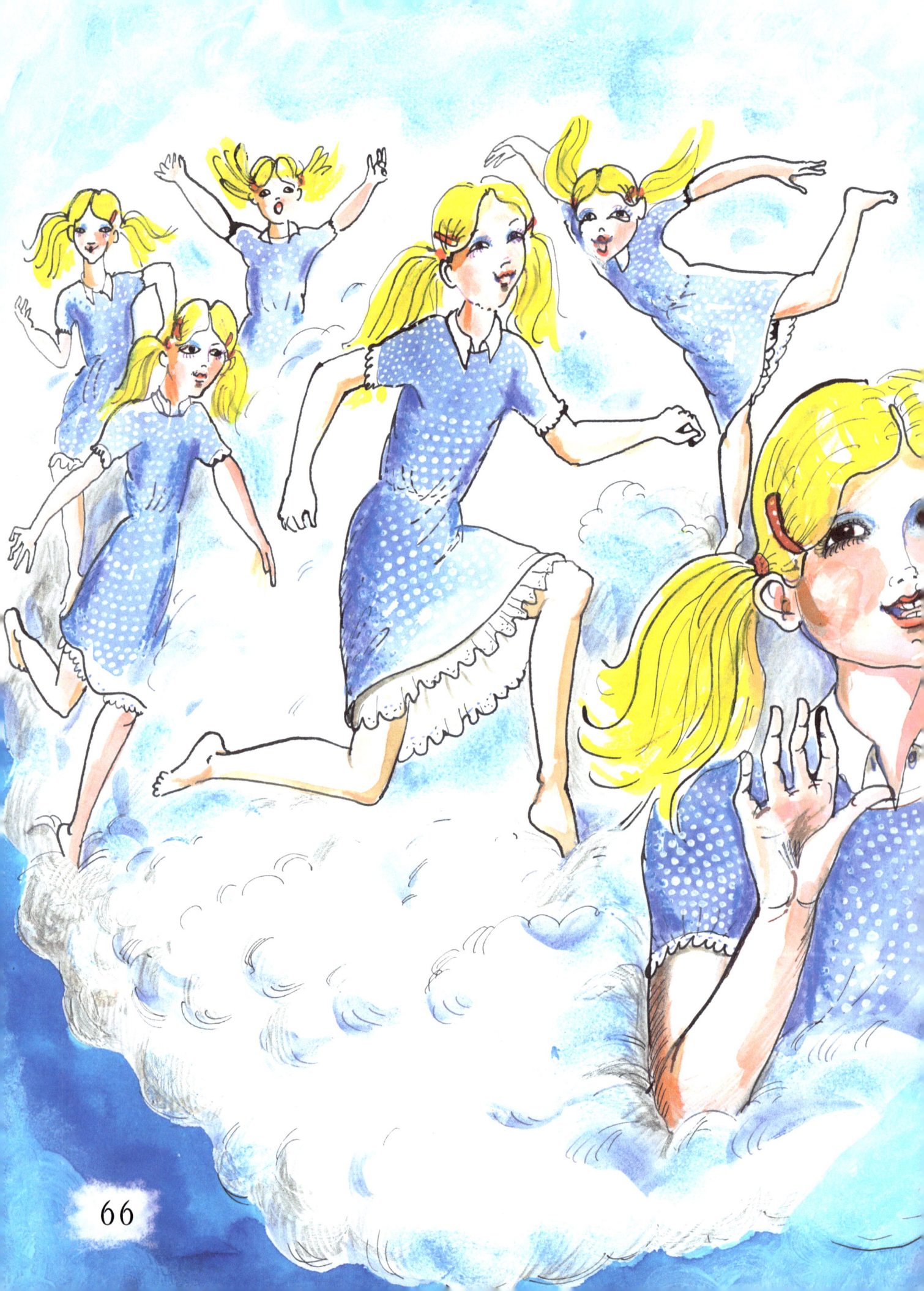

— "I flew over the clear waters of the beautiful blue lake, but al
I could see was a reflection of my Self looking back at me. It
was so wonderfully wonderful."

— "I felt brave and bright and very, very happy; and it
was like I loved everything. It was like my Happy Place
had grown and grown to fill everything in the whole
wide world."

"I flew high up to the clouds, and I didn't even
get tired."

— "I bounced from one cloud to another like tram-
polines with my hair almost bouncing off my head.
It was so much fun."

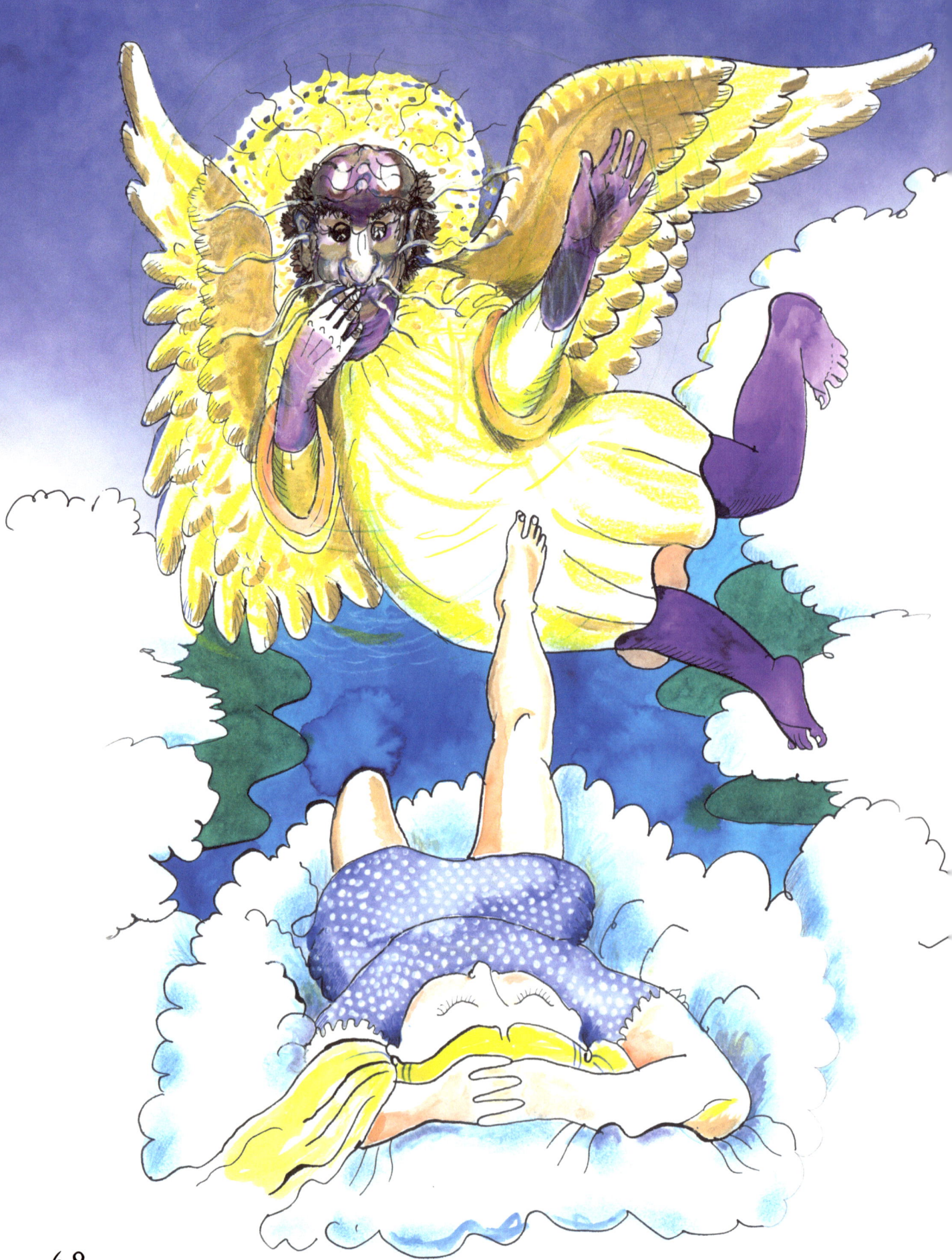

— "Then I lay on my back on a big billowy white cloud and looked straight up into the blue sky beyond the clouds."

— "And you know what? I saw the most lovely angel floating by. He had wide feathery wings of light and glowing strands dangling from his teeth that looked a lot like strings of spaghetti made of angel light. He waved and blew me a kiss as he floated up beyond the clouds and out of sight."

— "Then I rolled over on my tummy and peeked over the edge of the cloud, and do you know what I saw? I saw the beautiful blue lake with the long, long bridge going all the way over to the land of Nothing. Most of all, I saw all of you standing by the other end of the long, long bridge; and you all looked so very, very sad."

— "So I flew down to see what was the matter, and now I am here."

— "I see you are all very happy and that makes me happy, too."

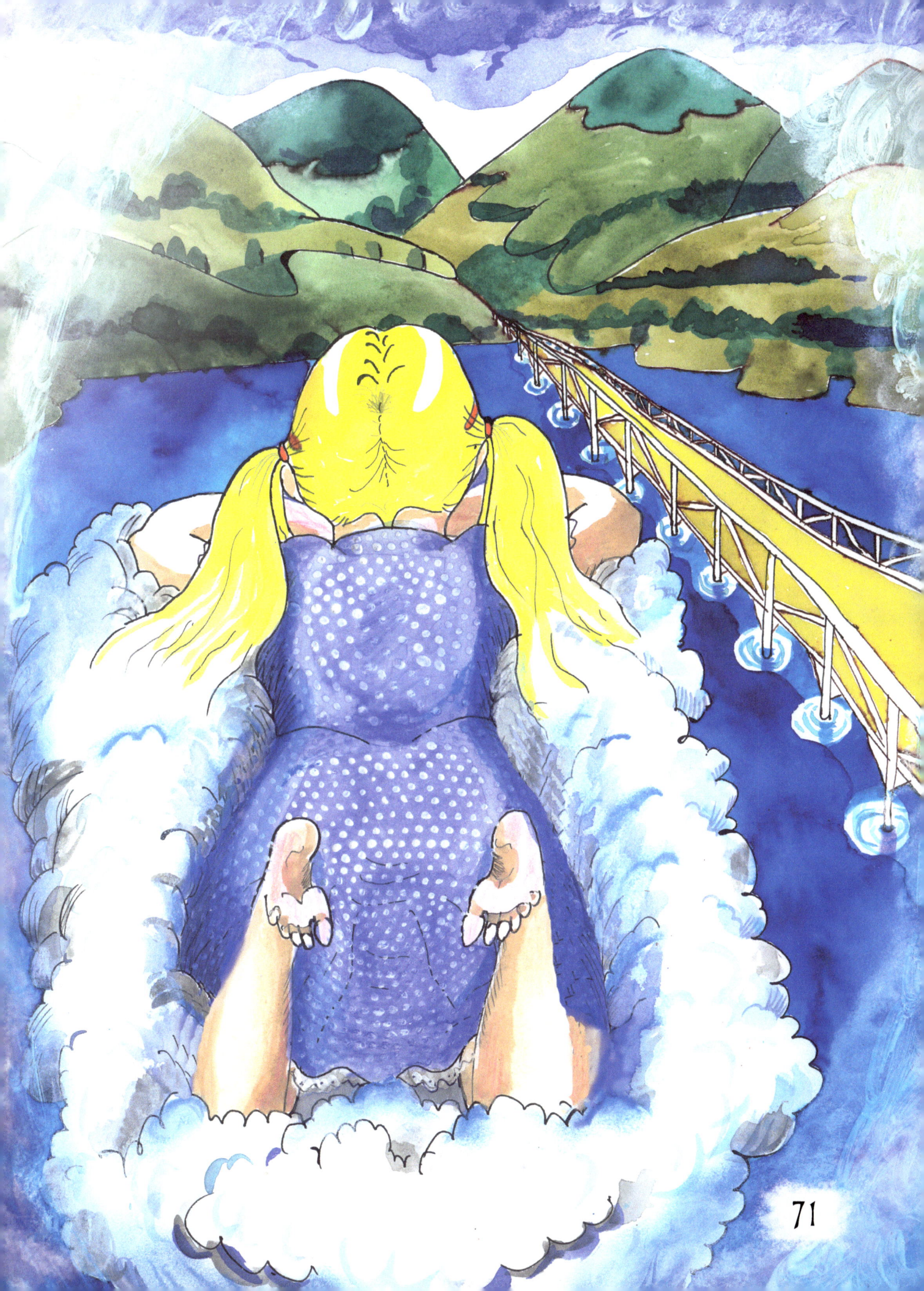

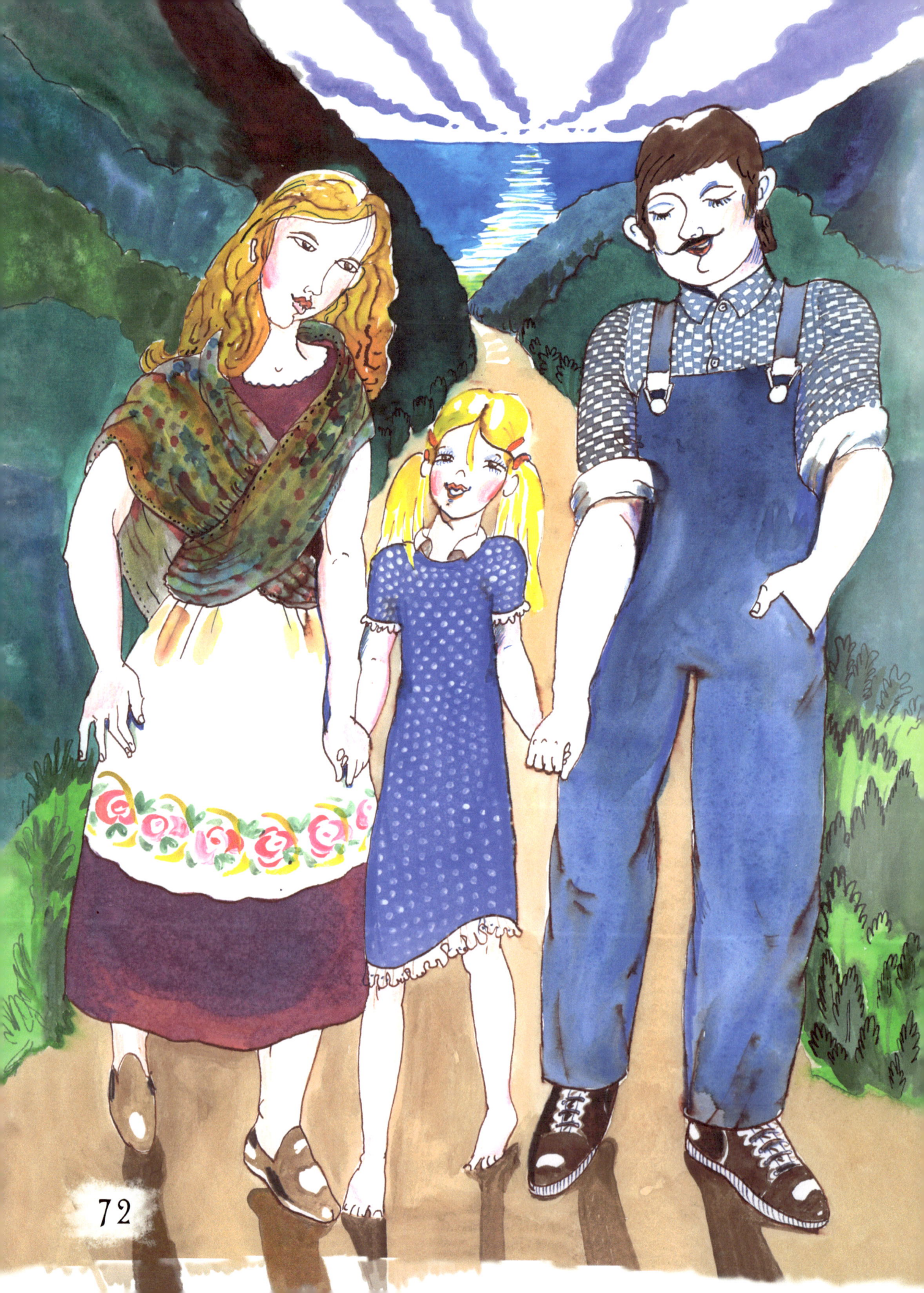

All the townspeople started back to their village on the other side of the hill. Sweet Little Martina held her parents' hands as she walked.

She looked lovingly up at her mother and then her father; and when she saw them both at the same time, a deep, unending love rose up in her heart. Her love engulfed her parents, and when it spread to all the people of the busy little village, they became happy without needing to be so very busy.

Sweet Little Martina walked with her mother and father back to the peaceful little village, and they all lived happily ever after.

Back by the beautiful blue lake next to the long, long bridge at the very spot where Ego the Ogre's tear fell in the dust, there grew a single sunshine daisy.

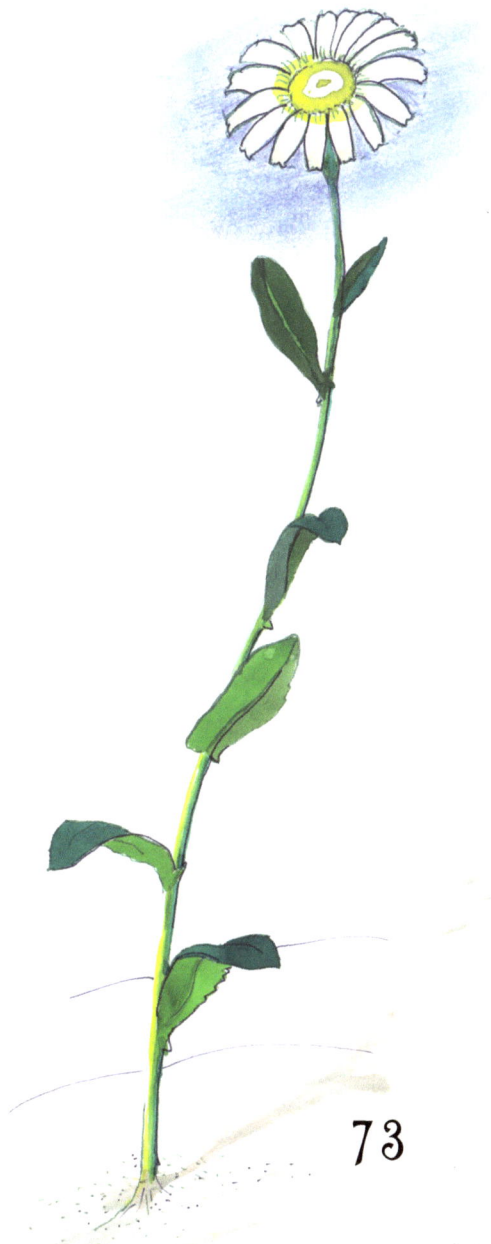

Readers who bought "Martina and the Ogre" also purchased:

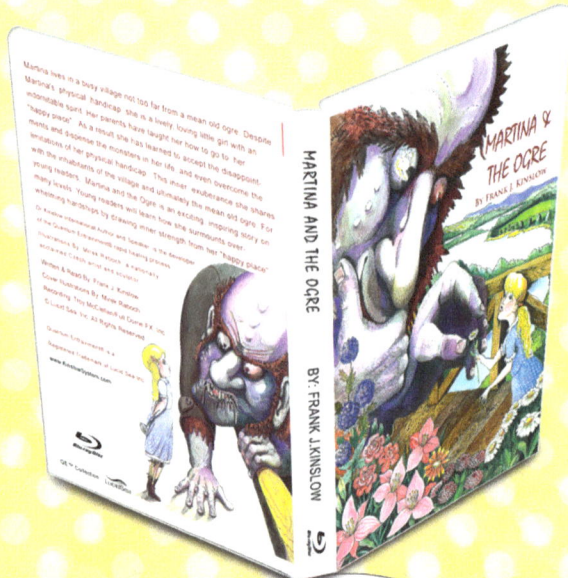

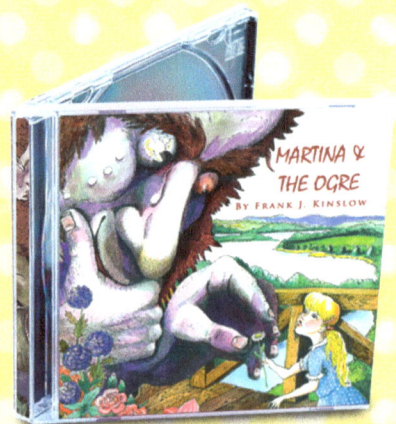

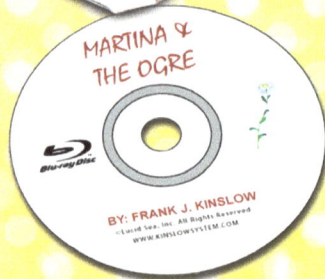

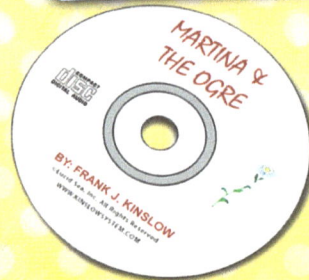

Martina & The Ogre
Blu-ray Disc

Martina & The Ogre
CD

Narrated by Frank Kinslow

Visit our Website at **www.MartinaandtheOgre.com**

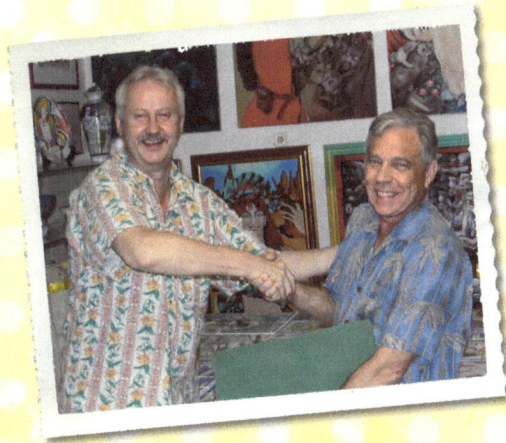

Frank Kinslow (above right) is an international best-selling author who, as a child at his mother's knee, listened enthralled as she fabricated fantastical tales about Frank, his friends and his family. Frank has inherited his mother's talent and writes in a friendly, conversational tone that makes the reader feel as if they were sitting comfortably together by a fire in their own living room. Through his characters, Frank gently confronts the reader with the challenges of life, answering them with wit, wisdom and humor. Frank lives in Sarasota, Florida with his wife Martina.

Mirek Raboch (above left) was born into an artistic family in Teplice, Czech Republic, in 1953. He has been the recipient of several national awards for painting, his first achieved when he was only seven years old. Raboch's paintings are well known for their rich color, action, and detail delighting children and adults the world over. He retired from teaching art to disabled children and now devotes fulltime to painting and sculpture. He resides in South Bohemia with his wife and two children, both of whom carry on the family's artistic tradition.

www.ingramcontent.com/pod-product-compliance
Lightning Source LLC
Chambersburg PA
CBHW041543260326
41914CB00015B/1533